Every Day We Are Killing Cancer

Heather Jose

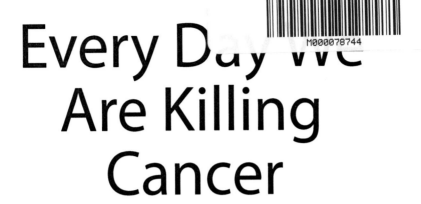

Read The Spirit Books

an imprint of
David Crumm Media, LLC
Canton, Michigan

For more information and further discussion, visit
www.EveryDayWeAreKillingCancer.com

Cover art and design by
Rick Nease
www.RickNeaseArt.com

Published By
Read The Spirit Books
an imprint of
David Crumm Media, LLC
42015 Ford Rd., Suite 234
Canton, Michigan, USA

For information about customized editions, bulk purchases
or permissions, contact David Crumm Media, LLC at info@
DavidCrummMedia.com

Contents

Foreword

THE BOOK YOU are about to read is a glowing example of victory in the face of uncertainty, a purposeful path in the midst of chaos and a tale of a mother's love for her daughter and family that kept her steadfast and focused in what would be the battle of and for her life! In this book, Heather Jose recounts every step and every emotion of her amazing journey. I can tell you that you will find this to be a great gift of incredible insight—an inspiring companion for you or a loved one facing cancer. This riveting story and the information contained within will serve both the newly diagnosed and those who are veteran survivors.

For me, seeing Heather for the first time was different than meeting most of the patients that had her same profile. She was an upbeat young woman who wore a bright blue bandana on her head and had an amazing smile. Heather was full of life and surrounded by family who loved and supported her. I thought to myself that she was much, much too young to fit the mold of someone who was battling stage IV breast cancer.

Heather had been through a lot, yet you would never know it by looking at her. I could see already that breast cancer, for

Heather, was going to be a mere speed bump in the road of life as she was determined not to let it define who she was, nor stand in the way of the best years that lay before her. This young woman was motivated, engaged and ready to partner in her own health—all, according to research, essential attributes of a cancer survivor.

Both in my personal and professional life, breast cancer is a familiar foe. I lost a great-grandmother, grandmother and mother all to breast cancer and know firsthand how devastating the disease can be. Make no mistake about it: Breast cancer and the treatments to tackle advanced stages of it are no walk in the park. A great percentage of the cancer patients that I've had the honor of helping with their nutrition came to me with advanced breast cancer. Some lived, some didn't. Some tolerated treatment and many really struggled through it. But the good news is that over the years, I've seen several people, like Heather, who were dealt a bad hand but still persevered and even thrived post-diagnoses. I've seen patients who chose to let their diagnosis be a launching point for a renewed quest for wellness and personal achievement.

Often, newly diagnosed patients are presented with pamphlets that offer general information about their disease, treatment options and their side effects that are typically over-generalized, impersonal and bleak in nature. Receiving the news that one has cancer is bad enough, but if that news is not accompanied with tailored messages of critical next steps infused with hope, the level of duress and even outcomes, can be negatively affected. Though this was initially the case for Heather, fortunately for her, she had family and friends who helped get her the answers she needed to properly battle cancer. Heather not only had great support but also chose to be an active participant in her own care. She utilized mind-body techniques, incorporated tailored nutrition and supplementation and engaged in physical care that helped minimize side effects of therapy and built up her strength and improved her response to treatment. So many patients are told to either not worry about changing their diet and lifestyle for the better or to wait until after treatment if they are going to do so, though evidence-based research refutes this still common and misguided bit of advice. Being engaged in one's care versus being a passive recipient can make all of the difference in the world in the quality of life one experiences during treatment and its outcome.

The good news is that beating breast cancer is becoming more commonplace. Strides in medical science, early detection, better treatment modalities and a greater understanding of the importance of incorporating adjunctive care like good nutrition into a treatment plan is making a substantial difference in survival rates. But so much more can be done and needs to be done. And having a personal companion like *Every Day We Are Killing Cancer* that can relate to what you or a loved one are going through and provide those essential words of hope can be the most important "medicine" in that critical time period after receiving the "news". You are not alone. You have a trusted friend in Heather.

—David W. Grotto, RD, LDN, nutrition expert
and author of *101 Foods That Could Save Your Life*

If You Are …

- *A survivor,* I want you to know that you can make a difference. It is your body. I would encourage you to think about your strengths and build a plan from there. You might be a great prayer-warrior, a fantastic list-maker or a dedicated workout person. Start from there and do something. It is your job to take the lead in this journey. Find people who can support you.

- *A caregiver,* I want you to know that you have a crucial role to play in your loved one getting well—however, you can't do it for them. They have to make that decision and they have to commit themselves. I have seen many, many well-intentioned caregivers trying to do more than the sick person wanted. You can support, but they have to *do*. As you read the Snapshots from my team, you'll see that they found ways to support me without coddling me.

- *A healthcare professional,* I want you to know (and I am very passionate about this), that your words matter. As patients, we are watching your every move, hoping for a little bit of encouragement. You have the ability to change our outlook for good or for bad. Even if the outcome is bad, there is always a place for hope. Please realize that we are people first, patients second. We want you to understand that we have families and dreams just like you. Often, our dreams hinge on the words you have to say. We are not just a block of time on your schedule. Forgive us for being anxious; we think you would be, too. We know you are busy, but it doesn't take any more time to do things in a positive way.

Preface

A Very Bad Day

IF YOU HAVE ever had a crisis, we have something in common. I never could have guessed what was about to unfold as I went in for a checkup—but I am getting ahead of myself.

As you begin this book, keep in mind it has a happy ending. It starts off pretty tragically and scary, but the outcome is good. It has been well over a decade since I found out that I had stage IV cancer. For most hearing that news, it sounds like a death sentence. I was 26.

I know the power of hope, and I will do all that I can to promote it. This book is not a how-to and there are no magic potions listed. I do know that each of us can make an impact, so why not start there. When I was diagnosed and looking for inspiration, it was so hard to find. That is why I wanted to share my story with you. If you read this and feel as though you can make a difference for yourself or someone else, I will have succeeded.

I am an ordinary woman. I say this because I want you to know that I believe that each of us has the ability to triumph over crisis. A crisis is often the catalyst to becoming the very best version of you. The opportunity to shine appears often, yet it is up to us to seize the chance to grow, to hope or to inspire others. I have no doubt that it is within all of us to do these things.

It is important to point out that I didn't walk into cancer with any special knowledge or information that would have helped me prepare for it. I had to learn quickly; to surround myself with good people; and draw on my own strengths. Each of us will do it differently, but the ability to succeed is there.

Just as I am not the person that I was when I underwent treatment, the world of breast cancer has changed too, in the last decade. The treatments that I decided on may not be the best anymore. The important thing is that the treatment that you choose is right for you and that you participate.

What started out as a collection of letters to my baby girl, grew into this book. After writing its first version, I realized I had not gone through this alone. I have included some thoughts and reactions written by my friends and family. Despite the fact that they were not diagnosed, they *were* along for the ride.

Though it was cancer that was the stimulus for change in my life, I know that there are many other factors out there that can set the ball in motion. I believe, more than anything, that how we handle challenges determines who we become.

Here is my story.

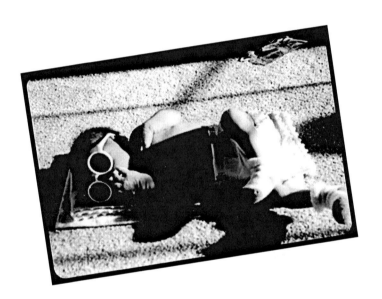

CHAPTER 1

A Routine Visit with Meredith

Sydney Bs,

I am going to rock your world when I am the one who is supposed to protect you from all the evils of the universe. I'm sure that you can't understand this at 14 months old, but I'm afraid you're going to feel the effects. You see, Mommy has this terrible thing called cancer, and it's threatening our time together. I love you, Chunks, and I thought I'd better write it all down. I remember the first time I saw your tiny toes. I couldn't believe how perfectly formed they were, and yet they were so small. Now you are a precious gift toddling around my house. You have this wild blonde hair (Where did you get blonde?) that sticks up no matter what. I love it. It completely suits you. I don't know how to prepare you for what is to come other than to promise that I'll take good care of you. People keep telling me that you won't even remember this. I have to say, that scares me more than anything right now.

Yours,

Mommy

IT STARTED WITH a lighthearted, routine visit to see Meredith. Meredith had gone to medical school with my older brother, Troy, and he referred me to her when I called to tell him I was pregnant. We had all gone through the pregnancy and delivery together. I will always remember Meredith in the birthing room announcing, "It's a girl! Sydney, right?" I was still in a daze and she had remembered the names we had chosen for a girl and named our baby.

I hadn't seen her since my six-week post-delivery checkup. She was more than a doctor, she was a friend. My husband, Larry, my 14-month-old daughter, Sydney, and I had all gone to my checkup so we could chat with Meredith.

So there we were in the exam room, marveling over Sydney's growth, commenting on Meredith's own pregnancy. I told her that I was there for my yearly checkup, but that I also had this nagging pain in my sternum that seemed to come and go. As soon as my top half was exposed, the questions about my left breast began. Meredith asked if the nipple had always been retracted. I answered no and redirected her to the pain in my chest.

"It feels muscular," I said. "Do you think it's from carrying my bags all the time?" I was working as an occupational therapist for a school system. Part of my everyday routine was carrying toy-laden bags in and out of elementary schools. Everyone could always tell who the school therapist was. We were the one carrying all the bags. They often weighed 50 pounds or more.

I went on to explain that the pain would go away with Tylenol, but I wanted to know why it was hurting. On a scale of 1 to 10, I ranked the pain a 4, nothing serious, just bothersome. It had been there for a while though, probably since the summer months.

Meredith continued to focus on my breast and after a few more questions asked if I would mind a colleague coming in to take a look. I agreed. After a quick look and a brief consultation with her in the hall Meredith came back in. I was ready for an explanation.

"Isn't this normal? All of my friends said that their breasts changed dramatically throughout pregnancy. I didn't think it was something I should be concerned about."

"It's probably nothing," Meredith said, "But I want to make sure."

"What could it be?" I asked, wanting a straight answer.

"A cyst, a benign tumor, or," with hesitation because she didn't want to tell me, "it could be cancer."

Cancer? Me, with cancer? I didn't even know what cancer was! I wasn't sure if I should be worried.

"Maybe it's one of those other things," she said.

We proceeded to pack up and go home while Meredith set up appointments to figure this whole thing out. By the time we arrived home we had convinced ourselves that we could handle it, and then we would move on.

No one ever has time to be sick. The week before I had resigned from my job to take a similar one closer to home. It would mean less driving and I would be working in our home school district, where my husband was a high school teacher and head football coach. I was excited about the prospect of working with people who lived in my community, getting to know them on a professional level, as well as becoming familiar with the elementary school that Sydney would attend one day. How would my future employer feel about this? I didn't even have a relationship established yet.

Besides the job thing, how could I have cancer? I am not atypical, and 26 year olds don't get breast cancer. I grew up in a small, uneventful town in southern Michigan. I am a middle child, the only sister to my older brother, Troy, and younger brother, Josh. We lived a normal life, my mom a computer programmer, my dad a biology teacher at the high school that we all attended. I had done well there, graduated and gone on to college to be an occupational therapist. While in college I met my husband at a YMCA camp where I was working in the summer. Six months after graduation from college we married and two years later Sydney was born. My life had always just rolled along, small ups and downs, but in the scheme of things, nothing extraordinary.

There is nothing like a life filled with small incidentals. A life where your biggest worry is the next positive changes in your life and the world is at your fingertips. I wish I knew that then.

Snapshot: Josh, Heather's Younger Brother

"I found out about Heather's cancer from my mom. I was a freshman in college and it was finals time, so she waited until I finished to tell me the news. I was overwhelmed, scared and even cried for a little bit. I went to my room and prayed. I remember thinking that she was probably the strongest one of all of us and if anyone could beat cancer it would be her. From that point, I didn't really look back.

"I always felt like Heather could beat it. I know now that I didn't really comprehend it. My goal was to not treat her any differently than before all this, since everyone else was. I hope I succeeded.

"Heather was strong and stubborn which was helpful, but there was also a will to win despite the odds. I've come to believe that if you can have a good support network, a strong faith, and a will to live, you will probably have a pretty good crack at it, regardless of what the doctors are saying.

"I think Heather's cancer created a stronger bond that no one talked much about in our family. It made us realize that life was precious. This was true for all of us. This was also when I decided that it was important to say 'I love you' every time I'd talk to them. I still do this to friends and family.

"Our dad was stoic, almost unflappable. I think it was killing him, but he wouldn't let his guard down. Mom had always been strong, but this rattled her. Then she buckled down and did what she had always done. She got us through.

"I went back to school after the holiday break and so I was disconnected from much of what was going on. My parents would come to school and watch me play hockey. Afterwards we would go out to eat. We didn't talk about Heather or her cancer. I felt like they were living with it 24/7 so I could give them a break. I wanted to keep things normal for them if I could. I think this carried me for the next couple of years. My job was to stay the course for my parents and family. I did that.

"While I'm not sure Heather would agree, I think I look at her cancer as a blessing. We are all different. While Troy and I didn't discuss it much, it made us realize how important it was to stay in touch. It helped us all to make an effort to connect. We try harder than we might have before.

"It's amazing what Heather's story has done to bond people. I have told it so many times. Especially since cancer is everywhere and it continues to happen. For me to be able to sit down and tell people a story that starts out with the worst possible scenario and share the outcome is a great thing. I've seen the impact it can have on people. That is a good thing."

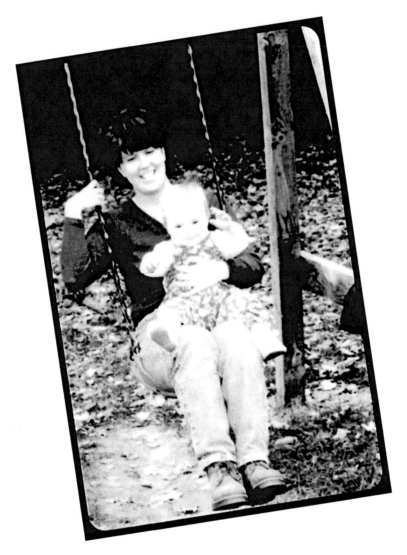

CHAPTER 2

A Normal Day

Sydney Bs,
So many things to talk about with you. I have so many dreams for you. Seeing you grow, hearing you say new words. Watching you become more than just my daughter, becoming my friend. I keep thinking that everything is going to be okay and then the fear sweeps in again. You make me feel better just by being you these days. You need me to help you grow. Doesn't the cancer know that? I'm going to fight with everything I've got, Hon. I'm going to watch you grow up.
Mommy

THE TESTING BEGAN the very next day about an hour south in Grand Rapids where Meredith was based. She had set up a series of procedures that would take much of the day. Larry and I found ourselves waiting for a mammogram, still not really believing any of this. As we dropped Sydney off with our neighbor Beth that morning, she told me that it was nothing and that everything would be fine.

The mammogram tech that escorted me into the exam area told me that I was awfully young to have breast cancer. It was absolutely surreal to be doing these tests that I associated with women much older than myself. I was getting an education quickly, learning the ins and outs of the mammogram, an ultrasound, and ultimately a biopsy. In between tests Larry and I sat in a series of waiting rooms and said little.

I ended my first day of testing in a small exam room having a biopsy done. The procedure was to insert a needle and try to extract liquid. Liquid is good. It means that it is probably a cyst, and certainly not cancer. A resident was doing the test, with his boss looking on. I should have taken my cue from the older doctor when he asked his resident if he would like him to perform the procedure.

"No, no," the resident answered, "I can do it."

The needle was unable to extract any liquid. They moved on to the next procedure where a sample of the cells was taken from various parts of the lump. This is done with a jagged type of needle, with a hollow core. As we were getting started Meredith came in, more for reassurance than anything else. I was glad to see a familiar face.

The procedure was painful and prolonged by the inexperience of the resident who had to do it repeatedly as he was unable to get what he needed. By the end of the procedure, I was lying on the table sobbing silently with tears rolling down my temples as I waited for them to leave. Meredith, standing at the end of the table, was touching my ankle saying she was sorry. I felt that life as I knew it had been taken away.

As we traveled home again, it felt as though it couldn't be true. I didn't think a perfectly healthy young person could just go to the doctor and find out that she had cancer. I didn't know how to handle any of my new thoughts about cancer. I still didn't have any answers, so I just went on, struggling to maintain an emotional balance.

I went to work the next day having regained my composure with the help of my husband. I even told some of the people that I worked with about the biopsy, confident that it would come back benign. Silly me.

It isn't just on television that people's lives are changed with one phone call. It happens all the time. Sometimes the phone calls bring changes we welcome. Other times, they change history. This was one of those.

Larry and I had just gotten home from work when the call from Meredith came. I answered the phone and she asked me if Larry was home too. When I answered yes, she asked if we could both get on a phone. At that point the shaking began—the uncontrollable tremble of fear.

"It's cancer," she said.

I was sitting on the side of my bed, on the quilt that had been made for us by my friend's mom for our wedding. My husband, on the cordless, came in to sit beside me.

There is something inside a person that takes over when the rest of you is falling apart. Without digesting the diagnosis, I asked what we would do next.

Meredith began to tell of the procedures.

"We'll need to do testing to find out how far it has gone," she began. She talked of speaking with a surgeon and an oncologist. We talked about telling my older brother, Troy, currently a flight surgeon in the Air Force, and having him in on decisions, even though he was miles away in Texas. At the end of the conversation Meredith told me that she knew yesterday, but she thought it might be better to give us one more normal day.

Larry had to make the toughest phone call of his life that night. He called my mom to tell her that I had cancer while I sat next to him on the couch and listened. I couldn't do it. I don't know why. I tell my mom everything, but I couldn't tell her this.

It was Thursday, December 10, 1998.

The next week was a wild mix of emotions. I felt caught between worlds as I tried to finish up things at my job when it was the last thing on my mind. My boss wanted to know when my reports would be ready to turn over to the person taking my place. Even after an explanation of my diagnosis, she wanted to know how I was going finish if I wasn't coming in to work. We were on the phone, as I sat on my living room floor with papers all around me, trying to sort things out. I was shocked at the insensitivity, but it was a quick lesson that the world goes on even when your life is falling apart.

My days were scattered. Some were spent at work, a couple were spent with follow-up tests, and all of them were spent fretting.

We then made our trip to meet with the doctors. One of the first doctors I met with was a surgeon, a nice middle-aged man who was talking on the phone with my brother, Troy, as I came into his office. I learned that surgery would likely be the first step to remove the tumor that measured 5 centimeters. I also learned that 5 centimeters was huge, in terms of tumors. He taught me about the stages of breast cancer and quoted survival statistics at each stage. By the time he got to stage IV he shook his head and said those statistics weren't so good.

The doctor then gave me pamphlets to read about cancer. You get diagnosed with a life-threatening disease and you get pamphlets. It's almost funny if you really think about it. The brightly colored pamphlets were about cancer, chemotherapy and radiation. I found the information inside dark and discouraging.

After leaving his office, Larry and I went back to the hospital to meet Meredith and her husband, Chad, also a doctor. They wanted to pray with us, and along with two other doctors, we found a quiet conference room on an upper floor of the hospital.

I had never prayed like that before, even with a lifetime of Sundays at church under my belt. It started with a verse read by

Chad. Then, with me sitting in a chair in the middle, everyone placed a hand on me. They prayed for complete healing and for protection for our family and me. They prayed for strength and direction, for good doctors and long life. It was deeply touching to have strangers pour their hearts out to God on my behalf.

We left that night feeling a bit better, a bit more prepared to fight.

I ended my first week of having cancer with yet another trip to Grand Rapids. This time I was having a bone scan, the big test to determine whether or not the cancer had spread to my bones. If there was cancer in any bones or organs, I would be stage IV. Of course, we still held hope that it wasn't that serious, that I was still in the "good" percentages the surgeon had spoken of.

For the scan I laid on the table in one of those ridiculous hospital gowns that three of my closest friends could have fit into with me. The surface was chilly and uncomfortable, although its design reminded me of a tanning bed. With the top closed down, you could lay your head to the side and watch all sorts of people scurrying around. There was no privacy. The machine itself was in a cubicle off a main hallway in the hospital. The tech that was administering my test didn't even bother to pull the curtain.

I was edgy before we got started. It was late in the afternoon and the scan was running behind. I still had to get to my first meeting with an oncologist, and I wasn't sure that we would make it. I had also been sitting in a room full of pregnant women as I waited. Whoever decided that it was a good idea to put women with cancer and pregnant women together had clearly never been in my shoes. They sat there and rubbed their bellies; I sat there and wondered how much of my life would be salvageable after cancer.

After my scan finally finished, the tech said, "We'd like you to go to X-ray to have some pictures done."

"No," I said, "I've already been there. I need to get to my oncology appointment."

"I know," she told me. "We'll let them know that you'll be a little late; we need some more pictures."

"Is there something wrong?" I asked, wondering if the shaking was from fear or cold.

Without answering she told me that x-ray was down the hall on the left.

Oh my God was all I could think as I walked out to Larry, the familiar tears welling up in my eyes. I was quite a sight I'm sure, standing in my enormous gown, holding the back shut with one hand and telling him in a quivering voice that they wanted more x-rays.

"OK," my tower of strength said. "It's OK. Maybe they just didn't get what they needed."

"Or maybe it's everywhere!" I burst out and then began to crumple into him.

Slowly I told him that I could see the screen during the test, that I saw a bunch of spots in different places. I didn't know what they were, but I had a pretty good guess. He gathered me up and held me for a minute, rubbing my back, running his fingers through my hair. He let his touch be my comfort, knowing there were no words for this situation that we were in. When he knew I was recovering, he asked if I was ready. I gave him a nod and off we went, down the hall and to the left.

This tech was a politician too, smiling when he thought it was appropriate, avoiding all of my questions and favoring small talk instead. He ushered me back into his room, big and cold with metal gleaming all around. I asked him about the views he was taking and after a few vague non-answers on his part I realized he wouldn't talk about what I wanted to talk about. Clamming up, I turned when he told me to and waited for the okay to put my clothes back on and regain just a little of my dignity.

I wondered if the downward spiral was ever going to end as we drove to the oncology appointment.

We arrived at his office late, with films in hand. After giving them to the receptionist we took a seat in the large waiting room. I don't recall any conversation. What was left to say?

After a while Larry and I were put in an exam room and the doctor appeared. He was taller than us, and he seemed to tower over me as I sat on the table. His tone was somber and a bit angry. He was difficult from the start, wanting to know if Meredith had told us the results of the bone scan. We explained that the scan had just been done, and then we came directly to him. After hearing that, he left us in the exam room and went to call Meredith, we found out later.

A few minutes passed and he reappeared, telling us that this wasn't his job, that my doctor should be telling me the results of my tests. By this time, I was completely frazzled though my outward appearance was one of unshakable composure. After a bit more hemming and hawing he began painting his dismal picture, still irritated that he was the one giving me the news.

"The cancer, I'm afraid, is in your bones. Once it leaves its primary site and begins to travel, it's quite difficult to control." He glanced up and went on, "You need to get your affairs in order." There was a brief pause and he added, "We can try some chemo, but I won't make any promises."

It hit me that he meant I had stage IV cancer. It had progressed so far that the percentages were dismal enough to make the surgeon I had met just shake his head rather than quote them to me. Now they were talking about me.

I'll never forget my next words, nor will Larry, as he was feeling as though he had been punched in the stomach. He couldn't believe how evenly I fired them out.

From my spot on the exam table I looked down at the doctor sitting in a chair.

"I'm 26 years old and that's the best you can do for me?"

He nodded his head slowly. He thought that was the best he could do. He did know of a colleague who was doing this very experimental stem cell procedure that he might be able to call.

He thought it would be best that we begin chemotherapy as soon as he got back from his skiing trip.

SKIING!!! I was dying, and he had the nerve to tell me he was going skiing. I had never been so low. Never mind that he told me to get my affairs in order. Seriously? How many affairs does a 26 year old have?

He proceeded to show us the chemotherapy area and hand me some more pamphlets. I was getting quite a collection by now. He explained that the nurse that ran this area would call and set things up with me. We left the office to walk into a cold, dark night. It matched my thoughts perfectly. That night's ride home seemed to take hours.

There wasn't much to be said. I was defeated. We went home and I called my mom, telling her it didn't look good.

December 17, 1998 had become the worst day of my life.

Lying in bed that night I asked Larry if he was scared to be alone. His response broke my heart. "I'm not scared to be alone; I'm scared to be without you."

Snapshot: Larry, Heather's Husband

"My initial reaction in the doctor's office was shock. I had been hearing him talking out in the hall. He came in and said, 'get your affairs in order' and the rest was 'blah, blah, blah.' My mind went blank. I am sure a lot of things were going through my mind, but it all boiled down to: *Holy crap, what am I going to do? I am not qualified for this!*

"I couldn't think at the time. Heather started asking questions, even grilling the doctor. I don't think I spoke until after we left the office. I couldn't. I was mute.

"We got home. I don't even remember driving. I don't remember telling my parents, who had been watching Sydney, what had happened. I know we did. When we were alone, Heather asked if I would call her mom. I did. It was a short call with awful news and not many options.

"The next day, with Heather's encouragement, I went to school. It was the last day before the Christmas break. It wasn't real."

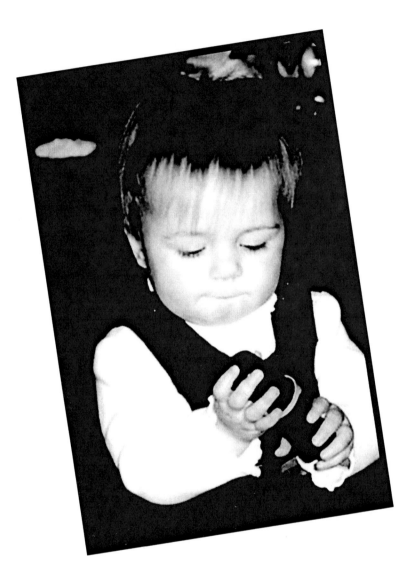

CHAPTER 3

Hope

Sydney Bs,

I can't wait to bake cookies with you. I want to be able to go shopping together, and watch you sing in a Christmas program. I am going to do those things; nobody else can be there like I can. How can cancer take away my time with you? Doesn't it realize you need me? I know you can't answer that; sometimes you just have to ask. Do you know how I met Daddy? It was at a summer camp where I was working. He came with Uncle Rob to chaperone kids. He wasn't much help though; as soon as we met he spent all of his time with me and my friend Katie. We enjoyed being together from the start; there is nobody that I would rather be with. I hope you find someone like that someday. I love you Syd.

Mommy

LARRY WENT TO work the next day, the Friday before Christmas break. He'd already missed a couple of days, and it looked as though he would be missing more. I stayed home with Sydney, moping, not knowing what to do. It was strange. I felt fine, but I was dying? I thought that's what the doctor told me yesterday.

I turned on the TV to try to take my mind off the craziness of my life. It only intensified it. How could people be clapping and cheering on *The Price is Right*? Didn't they know what was happening to me? I felt as though I couldn't fit into my own life anymore.

Sydney, having just celebrated her first birthday a few months ago, was becoming more of a little person each day. Thankfully, she seemed oblivious to all the changes in our lives. Her needs remained the same. In some ways that was comforting. She just expected me to take care of her.

My friend Marnie called mid-morning. Marnie was my PT (physical therapist) counterpart at work. She worked in the same schools as I did and saw a lot of the same kids. Marnie was the one who showed me around when I started, and we had developed a friendship as we worked together. We could talk for hours about anything and I found myself looking forward to the days we would be working in the same building on the same day. We were night and day in many ways. She's tall and willowy with blond hair and blue eyes, and I stand a stockier 5'5" with dark hair and hazel eyes. Marnie was in the band in high school. I was an athlete. There was an understanding between us even without words and we shared a mutual faith in God. This morning we cried together.

As our call began, I found myself sobbing about Sydney, "I've still got so much I need to tell her." I was sitting on the bottom step of the stairs, head down, feeling as though I would crumple into the floor. I had just seen a program where a dying mother made videos for her children. I wondered if I'd be doing the same.

Marnie, a mom of two angels of her own, replied, "I know, I know. We'll take care of that if we need to."

She gave me an honest answer, admitting to me that this was a serious battle that I was beginning.

She went on, "I am praying for complete healing. I haven't always done that in the past for others. I may pray for strength or for God's will, but this time I believe it is right to ask for healing." *Go, Marnie, go!*

Marnie's ability to pray for complete healing was a shot of hope to me. Most people I had encountered in the last week said the normal churchy kind of things like "God's will be done" or "God has a plan." My problem with those statements was that they felt like I was not going to make it. Marnie's claim for complete healing for me was a great thing. It told me that we knew we needed God's power, but that death didn't have to be the outcome.

Marnie gave me strength to carry on, and after a long conversation I decided to pack up Sydney and travel the 50 minutes of back roads to get to her house. Marnie had troubles of her own right then. Two days before my initial diagnosis she fell and broke her leg. The two bones below the knee snapped, both of them clean through. Marnie was housebound for a while, a virtual blessing in disguise. I needed her to be there for me. God saw to it that it happened. Had she not broken her leg, Marnie would have been running her normal life at mach 10.

Marnie's house was always a bit like a circus. This morning, when I arrived, her kids were running around while her mom was trying to get lunch together. Mike, her husband, came in to check on things and headed back to work on the farm where they lived.

The dining room was the center of her house and all the activity revolved around it. There was a constant motion of kids and daily life. It was nice to be engulfed in the sound of voices; it'd been too quiet at my house lately. Rather than feel awkward, at Marnie's you just got swept up into the motion. Before I knew it Sydney was entertained and Marnie and I were talking over a stir-fry dish that a friend had brought over to her, the invalid.

I told her about my visit at the doctor the day before and how horrible it was. I told her about calling my mom, who in turn called my brother, Troy. My mom told him this was not acceptable, and they needed to do something. Troy dropped everything in Texas and got to work being a big brother. Troy had always taken that job seriously. From the time we were little I knew that he would look out for me. Sure, we had our fights, but I never doubted Troy's devotion to me or my younger brother Josh.

I gave Marnie all the details on how Troy first talked with Meredith and they decided that their medical school alma mater, the University of Michigan, was the best place to start. Next, he called a doctor with whom he had worked and asked him who the best doctor was for fighting breast cancer. He was given the name of Dr. Sofia Merajver, and he proceeded to track her down in her lab.

While I was still at Marnie's, Troy called me and told me Dr. Merajver would be calling. He had given her all the information he had and she responded with, "She's a U of M patient." What she meant was that she felt that they could provide the best care possible for my disease, and that she wasn't scared by it. Within the hour my phone rang again—it was Dr. Merajver.

Her quiet voice, competing with all of the noise our kids created, made it difficult for me to hear everything. I stole away to a quiet room and began to answer her questions. They were not about the cancer; they were about my family, my life and me. We began talking about the different ways of killing cancer. After a lot of reassurance, Dr. Merajver gave me her home phone number and some instructions for the weekend.

"Start drinking green tea, eat lots of fruit and veggies and we'll start killing cancer on Monday."

On Monday? Not after Christmas? Not after skiing? No. We were already killing cancer; she just gave me the okay to fight.

I hung up the phone and walked out to Marnie, not quite believing it had all happened. *Her home phone number? Do doctors do that?*

It was the first glimpse of hope I'd seen in a week. Like a breath of fresh air it revitalized me, helped me to stand up straight and move forward. Dr. Merajver would never know how much that conversation mattered to me.

Still in shock, I began to tell Marnie about the conversation.

"She asked about me and my job. She wanted to know how old Sydney was. She asked about Larry and whether or not we had a good marriage. It was a long time before we even talked about the cancer. She's so much better than the first guy. I'm going on Monday."

Marnie just listened to me as I went on and on. She, too, was relieved to see a ray of hope.

The prayer that had been prayed that night with Meredith to bring the right doctor into my life had been answered. I was sure of it.

Still on a high from my conversation with Dr. Merajver, I decided I needed to live my life, whatever was left of it. We had tickets to an Amy Grant Christmas program for the next night. She was a favorite Christian artist that I admired. Larry and I were supposed to go with a group of people from our church. Marnie and her husband, Mike, were supposed to go, too. Mike had gotten tickets long before Marnie's spill on the front porch.

I knew I couldn't face a group of people yet. The reaction of the few people I had seen since my diagnosis was to cry, which made me cry. Since Marnie and I had already moved past that, I thought it might work to go to the concert together. We planned to meet at her house the next day.

The drive down to Grand Rapids for the concert was uneventful, but the conversation was difficult. It is hard to make small talk with someone who has just been diagnosed with cancer. Larry and Mike tried to talk about skiing, a common interest. I sat quietly and turned everything said into something about cancer. I wondered if I would ever plan a trip again; or if Larry would take them without me someday.

After dinner at the restaurant near the arena, we headed over to the concert. Larry and Mike had gone early and sweet-talked an usher into letting us into handicapped seating on account of Marnie's wheelchair. The seats were good, the music was good, but my ability to cope was not good. I listened with tears sliding down my cheeks. I couldn't fight off the thoughts of not seeing my daughter grow, of making my husband a widower before he turned 30, and of how everyone else at the concert was celebrating just another Christmas. Before long I was having a spectacular pity party while the others enjoyed the concert.

I had spotted our group from church soon after we were seated. They were way up high, to the left of the stage. The thought of facing them sapped the rest of my strength. I have never been great at handling other peoples' emotions. I had no idea what to do with their expressions of sadness. At the intermission, Larry asked if I wanted to go up to say hello. I didn't, but I went anyway. I walked the steps to the top and waited for the reaction. There were hugs and some talk of how much better our seats were. It was the idle conversation that I was becoming used to. I was discovering no one knew how to make this any better.

As we returned to our seats, Marnie said I looked as though a weight had been lifted from my shoulders. It was true. I had faced the first group of people I knew as "someone with cancer", and now I could face more. As the second part of the concert began, I actually found the strength to sing a little, my terrible voice right next to Marnie's beautiful one.

Snapshot: Marnie, Heather's PT Co-Worker

"Circumstances seem so crazy until you believe in the sovereignty of God. The week Heather was diagnosed with cancer is etched in my memory forever as one of those times when life seemed out-of-control crazy—until we were on the other side of it looking back.

"I was a busy mom working part-time, raising two preschoolers ages 4 and a half and 3, plus volunteering—a lot. It was a Tuesday morning and I was headed out to work with two or three bags on my shoulders and hot chocolate in my hand when I walked out the door to my waiting car already loaded with overnight bags as we were going to a hotel right after work for a conference where I had volunteered to sing special music at a breakfast meeting the next morning. As I stepped down onto the final frost-covered step, my foot slipped and I dropped to the ground. In the few seconds it took for the pain to register, I reached down and felt my lower leg and knew that it was broken. I was lucky the bone hadn't come through the skin. Fast forward two days and I am now stuck in a recliner in a long leg cast all the way to my groin, hurting and feeling sorry for myself when the phone rings. Heather says to me, 'Start praying, it's cancer.'

"How can a broken leg be a good thing? When it makes you immediately accessible to a friend with far greater concerns and needs. It is hard to be a support person to a dear friend fighting for her life against a vicious and unseen assailant, but I will forever be grateful for the winter I spent recovering from a broken leg and being available to listen, encourage, cry with, and pray for Heather whenever she called or I could get her to visit. I was given the precious gift of watching God work powerfully in Heather's heart, mind and body throughout her fight, but especially during those first few months. Because of that experience, my God is much bigger than He was before and my faith is much stronger."

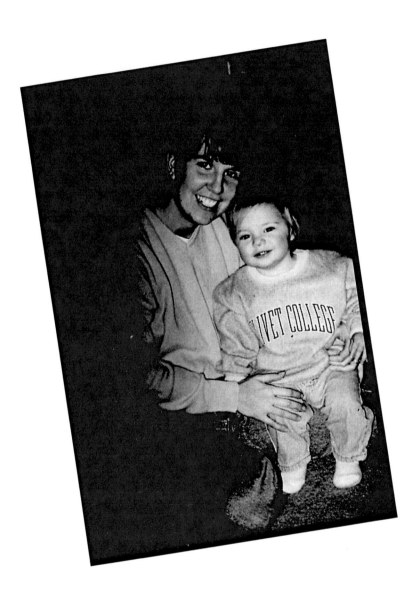

CHAPTER 4

Amaizin' Blue

Sydney Bs,

We make plans all of the time. We're going to do this and then that and on and on. I had made all those plans, and they were moving along rather smoothly. And then in a day it changes. That is why every day is so important. Every day you can make a difference in the way that your day goes. You can shrug off an angry person, or you can get angry too. You can make someone else's day by smiling. In this world that seems to be all about stuff, it isn't that at all. It's about people. There is nothing better than the sound of your all out belly laugh. I smile thinking of it. Or being on the couch, you, me and Daddy. That is it, heaven on earth. I treasure you more every day.

Loving you,

Mommy

EARLY THE FOLLOWING Monday morning Larry, my mom and I set out for Ann Arbor to find Dr. Merajver. Armed with maps from the Internet and directions that Troy had given us over the phone, we wound our way through the hills and curves and one-way streets of Ann Arbor to find ourselves in front of a rounded glass building tucked in behind the main hospital. As luck would have it, it even had its own adjoining parking ramp. As we pulled in, we were greeted with a computer-generated female voice welcoming us to the University of Michigan's Comprehensive Cancer Center. The name and building were impressive, and a bit intimidating.

Once inside, we began to learn the ropes. First and foremost, I needed a hospital blue card. On the main floor of the center we sat down with a receptionist who gathered all of our information about employment, insurance and next of kin. She then produced a plastic card in U of M blue. This card would be the first thing that everyone would ask for at every desk in the hospital. The card was used to convey just about everything, including what appointments were scheduled and what labs needed to be drawn. "Have you got your blue card?" had to be one of the most common questions asked on a daily basis.

Our next stop was about 50 feet to the left of the main reception desk. It was the blood draw station, a.k.a. the vampires. It is a respectful term; there is nobody better at getting blood than these people, even from disappearing veins. A woman asked for my card and told me she would call me when it was my turn. A chance to sit down gave me the opportunity to look around. It was a large space with lots of open air. The blood draw area separated itself with partitions rather than walls, allowing all the areas of the main floor to be separate and yet together. It was a cornucopia of textures and life that made me wonder. At various locations there were small, artful sculptures encapsulated in glass. The furniture was upholstered in a tweedy fabric, and chairs and love seats were gathered together in small groups to achieve a homey effect.

The people were the most amazing feature of what we saw. Young children with their parents, old people with their children. Some looked frightfully ill; others appeared as fit as marathon runners. It was hard not to wonder how cancer brought each of them here and if they would survive. I didn't feel as though I fit in with any of them. You could tell that many were regulars by the way they greeted and were greeted by the staff.

"How are you doing today?" followed by, "Wow, your hair is growing again!" It shocked me that this was normal conversation within these walls.

After a blood draw, where I wondered if they were going to drain me dry, I was sent upstairs to meet my doctor. Obviously they had lots of labs to run.

Mondays are Breast Clinic days at U of M and the waiting area, which could seat a lot of people, was packed. After signing in and leaving all of the films that I brought with the receptionist, I waited my turn. I had no expectations of being seen quickly as I knew I had been squeezed in. Once again I looked around, never knowing that so many people dealt with breast cancer. It took no time at all to also realize that I was easily younger than all of them. I don't recall any conversation between my mom, Larry and me. We were all lost in our own thoughts.

It took a while but my name was called, my vital statistics taken and we were all ushered into one of many examining rooms. Before long, Ginny strolled in, making me feel at ease instantly. Her title was Nurse Practitioner but her mannerism was that of my best friend's mom who I had known all my life. She was short with graying hair, an easy smile, and a concerned but confident tone. After giving her a synopsis of the last week, which had turned my world upside down, she left to go and get Dr. Merajver. It surprised me that she handled it all so easily. It was as if 26 year olds with stage IV cancer come her way all the time.

"Heather? I am Sofia Merajver. How are you doing?" I turned on hearing the familiar voice I had heard in my phone conversation. We were now face to face. She was "Sofia," not "Doctor Merajver." I was relieved.

I briefly introduced my mom and Larry and then we began to talk about the cancer. The discussion helped us to understand each other better. I made it clear that though I was really scared, I was going to fight and I needed someone to help me. Dr. Merajver told me that I was strong and that we had options. We could be aggressive in attacking the cancer or we could just try to extend my life and make me comfortable while the cancer took over.

"Cancer does not scare me," she said. "I see how it works. It can be tricky, but we will fight it."

I did not even hear the part about just trying to extend my life. I was singularly focused on getting rid of the cancer. I told Dr. Merajver that I had heard so much bad news that I only wanted to discuss moving forward at this point. I wasn't interested in knowing all of the places that the cancer had spread to in my bones. I told her that my husband and I had talked about it and agreed that if information like that was necessary for someone to know he would be the one. I knew it would only make me feel worse. I didn't need any more ammunition for negative thoughts.

In the short time that I had been dealing with cancer I had already felt how much negative thoughts impacted me. Ever since I had found out that the pain in my sternum was from the cancer, I analyzed every possible ache for another potential spot that the cancer was attacking. This was a huge drain on me emotionally. With Larry encouraging me, I trusted my instincts and decided to shut as much of the negative out as possible. This helped me gain control over a situation that had been snowballing since we heard the word cancer.

Dr. Merajver was okay with my philosophy but she said we needed to make sure that the cancer hadn't gone anywhere else, so she would order a few more tests—a CT scan of my brain, to be sure there was no cancer there; and an MRI to get a good look at all of my organs. The prospect of more tests made me shiver. Every test that I had taken since being diagnosed had been bad, revealing more cancer and grimmer chances. I wasn't sure I could handle much more. After all, less than two weeks ago my life was normal. On the other hand, how much worse than metastatic disease could it get?

We moved on to the next life change as the question of children was raised.

"You have a daughter, right?" Dr. Merajver asked, "Did you plan on having more?"

Larry and I looked at each other and then I mumbled that we didn't know.

My mom answered for us. "You had planned on having more than one child," she said.

"Yes," I answered. "We did."

She told us it would not be good for me to get pregnant, especially as I went through treatment. When I asked if it would be possible in the future, Dr. Merajver told me that we would wait and see. The drugs I would be using were powerful though, and she told me my chances of having viable eggs left were not good. Add to that a cancer that was hormone driven and we would never want to fuel it with all the hormones needed to carry a baby. In a few short moments, another plan for my future fell by the wayside.

My dream to have more children was replaced with killing cancer. It was now a fact, as much as stating that the sky is blue. This was a whole new ball game from my previous life. It was about facts and not feelings. No time to feel sorry. There were things to do.

We moved on to talk of the course of treatment that would be starting immediately and I began to learn the words that would become a regular part of my vocabulary. It was a world I knew nothing of and yet was engulfed in. Where were the days of idle conversation? Wow.

We spoke first of chemotherapy, and of the drugs which she felt would be the most effective. I would start with two drugs initially, Adriomyacin and Taxotere. Dr. Merajver instilled confidence in the drugs as she talked, leading me to believe they could take on anything. After four rounds of this regimen we could possibly do a stem cell transplant, a newer procedure which uses high-dose chemotherapy first and then stem cells to reintroduce life to my body. Surgery and radiation were also possibilities.

It was amazing, really. I felt as though I had more options than I might even need to take on the cancer. A couple of days earlier I didn't have any. I learned quickly what a difference a doctor makes. It wasn't just what she was doing in terms of medicine, it was the hope and confidence she instilled in me. Because of this I knew that I would use any time that I felt good to move forward and kill cancer. I became less of a victim and more of a partner because of her words.

Next was a physical examination. If she was shocked at the size of the tumor, I never knew. Instead, she reassured me that finding it would have been difficult, given the location behind the nipple and the changes with pregnancy and breast-feeding.

After the exam, Dr. Merajver left to get Kelly. I would soon discover Kelly was my "answer man." If I had a question, she had an answer. Kelly entered with an easy but professional manner. She looked to be in her 20s, a fit person with short auburn hair. Kelly exuded capability and after a quick introduction and a bit of joking with Dr. Merajver she walked me through the handful of prescriptions she held in her hand. First, there were drugs to help with nausea after the chemo. Next, Kelly asked if I could give myself a series of shots to help with my white blood count. Feeling tough, I answered yes, though I'd never done anything like that. Finally, there were the pre-medications to take before I came for chemo again in three weeks.

Kelly proceeded to give me phone number upon phone number so that I could always get in touch with her. No subject was off limits—from my sex life to my hair falling out. Kelly informed me that the hair would be gone two weeks to the day after my first chemo session. I had thought that would be the case. I had already cut it short so there would be less to fall out.

Before leaving the room to take me down to the infusion area to start my chemo, Kelly gave me a hug and said words that I will never forget. "You're my age; we're not going to lose you."

If you ever wonder if words matter, let me be the one to tell you that they do. Every single day.

In meeting with Ginny, Dr. Merajver and Kelly, I was given a lifeboat. I knew the sea was stormy but at least I had some way of trying to get to the shore. The talk of death was left with the doctor who was skiing right now. I had so much confidence in my new team. They were all more knowledgeable and approachable than I ever could have imagined. U of M prides itself on being "the leaders and the best." I didn't doubt that for a second. I understood a little bit more about the arrogance that surrounded U of M. They were willing to take on the most challenging situations; I felt they had earned it.

Snapshot: Dr. Merajver, Heather's Doctor at U of M

"I can recall taking the call in the lab where I was working on discovering breast cancer genes. It was Friday afternoon, I believe, and the person putting the call through said that it was a U of M graduate who urgently needed to speak to me about his sister who had breast cancer. I think I called him back a little while later. We spoke for about 20–30 minutes. He ran Heather's case by me and early on I knew, instinctively, that we (Heather and I) would be together for a long time. I noticed the sadness and resolution in his voice to find help in a place where he thought all doors would be open and where we would come up with something to do for his sister! I asked him for permission to call and if Heather knew he was talking to me. I told him to tell her I would call later. I finished the experiments I was doing and thought about what I would say, how I would approach the conversation and decided in my mind that I would simply tell Heather to dream of a life surviving this and that we would handle the rest together. I hope it came out that way.

"From the beginning, I admired Heather's positive attitude and perseverance; I thought she had excellent family and friends to support her; I felt everyone was positive and helpful in a way that made my job easier. Heather was always open to plans and suggestions for treatments and checkups. Together, we built a strong team to get it done! We are still going strong and making joint decisions the same way we did 14–15 years ago.

"It has been wonderful to get to know Heather and her family; to overcome all the obstacles so far; and to run a 10k together as a symbol of our bond and our pact to fight cancer every day."

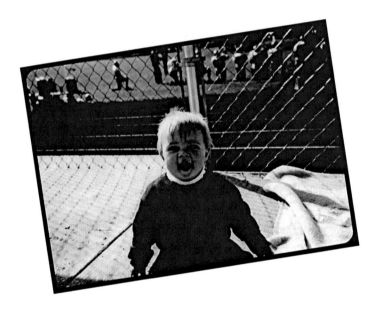

CHAPTER 5

Crossing Over

Sydney Bs,
There is nothing I want more than the chance to make memories with you and Daddy. I have great ones from being a kid myself. From spending hours riding my bike and playing with Christy to singing in the car and taking vacations with my family. I hope I can pass some of those on to you. It would be great if you could love Sarasota Sands the way that I love it. And if you can learn to camp, and explore cities, and well, there are so many things. Guess I'll just have to stick around and make it happen.
Love you,
Mommy

IT WAS A short walk down to the infusion area from Dr. Merajver's clinic. I was finding that everywhere we went the activity level was on high, an intermingling of separate doctors and services all together creating one loud hum. Having only seen the small infusion area at the first oncologist's office, I was amazed at the scene here. There was a large waiting area, once again full of people. Things looked a little more serious here. More bald heads, more hats, more people who looked frail, and some with masks.

When my name was called, we got a quick tour of the infusion area. The entrance was a large hallway with a well-stocked kitchenette on the right. There was a variety of drinks and snacks openly available to all during treatment. The hallway then opened up as it followed a circular path. Near the windows were reclining chairs, one after another. I realized that we were inside the rounded glass that I had seen from the outside. There were people resting in reclining chairs and getting their chemo, with family and friends sitting close by. At each recliner there was an IV pole with all sorts of bags hanging from it. It was a busy area, with nurses constantly moving about, yet very low-key. Some people were talking and watching TV, others sleeping. All were fighting cancer.

Off of the recliner wing, behind the kitchenette, was a smaller circle that had individual rooms with hospital beds in them. These were for the people who were really sick, or for the rookies like me. I was shown to a room with a view of the Ann Arbor hills and we settled in with me in the bed and Mom and Larry sitting alongside. We turned on the TV and chitchatted as we waited.

That is when I met my nurse Marlene. I can't recall a lot of nurses that I've encountered, but I will never forget Marlene. I liked her instantly, as did Larry and my mom. It can't be easy to put a family at ease during a first chemo session, but she did that for us, and we will always be grateful.

It began by inserting an IV in my arm and starting the fluids. Marlene put on her protective gear, including a gown and gloves, and then she hooked a bag of the Taxotere to my pole. She told me she would start it slowly. I was to tell her if I wasn't feeling well or if I felt like I couldn't breathe. As it went in, nausea immediately swept over me. It was accompanied with a heat that began in my arm and crawled up to my ears. Marlene was watching and backed off the Taxotere. I was having a reaction.

Up to this point, all I knew about chemo I had learned from TV or fictional books. It made a person throw up a lot. They lost their hair. Kelly had already told me that I would be losing my locks, so I assumed the throwing up part was also true. I thought the reaction I was having was normal. Marlene assured me that the intense heat and nausea weren't.

I believe there is such a thing as knowing too much. Along with not knowing where all of my bone mets (spots already attacked by cancer) were I also chose not to know all of the side effects of the drugs I was taking. The reasoning was the same. I did not want to be looking for things that were wrong or finding excuses as to why I shouldn't do something. My mom and husband assured me that they would know what the side effects were so that I could ask about anything unusual. They would know whether or not to be concerned. Therefore, I could convince myself of what was going right, instead of focusing on everything that could go wrong.

After taking more Decadron and Benadryl to stop my reaction, Marlene tried the chemo again. This time there were no problems, and in it flowed to find the cancer and destroy it. It took an hour and a half to do the Taxotere. When it was complete we moved on to Adriomyocin. Marlene told me they called it the "Red Devil" because it was red in color and so strong. I loved the name and the fact that it was tough as nails. My cancer didn't stand a chance. In five minutes it was in and I was done. We could leave.

I walked out of the cancer center looking the same as I did when I entered. However, I was not the same. A lot had changed in the time I was there. I now had some hope and a purpose: killing cancer. This was new. A small part of me still wanted to believe this was a bad dream. I knew this though: If cancer does one thing, it insures that your life will never be the same.

Upon arriving home, I felt ready to tackle the task of informing everyone about what was going on. I finally had a few answers and a plan as to how we would proceed. Our news had been spreading quickly and it seemed we were in the midst of uncomfortable conversations with virtually everyone. I felt like no one could say anything that seemed appropriate. Some people would say things like, "it will be fine" to which I wanted to scream: *REALLY? WHAT PART OF STAGE IV CANCER IS FINE?* Others would launch in to a discussion of someone that they knew who had cancer and more often than not it ended in death.

Note to self: Do not tell stories about dying to a person who is battling a life-threatening disease.

I think I reached a tipping point when a friend of Larry's called our house after having heard the news. I answered the phone and he quickly asked to speak with Larry. It was as if he didn't know who I was. I was a leper—untouchable and not to be spoken to. I felt a wall going up around me. It was devastating.

In truth, he was only one of a growing number that made me feel as though I was being placed outside of the world I lived in. So in an effort to save myself and help everyone feel more comfortable I wrote the first of what would be multiple letters.

> Dear Friends,
> I am writing this letter to tell you that we have a mountain to climb and we would appreciate your help. The past week has been amazing, but enlightening. On Thursday evening I got a call from my doctor to tell me that I have breast cancer. What a big word! We are in the midst of doing numerous tests and charting a course for treatment. It is definite that I will have chemo now, and will have a mastectomy later. We have all agreed that it will be treated aggressively, though it won't be

pleasant. Please don't feel sorry for me. Cry if you need to, I certainly do, but after that please decide to make a difference. We need your prayers. God says in James that if any of us are in trouble we should pray. Whether happy or troubled or sick, we should pray. We should call the elders of the church to pray and anoint the sick with oil, knowing that the person offered in faith will be well. If you wonder if you can make a difference we know that you can. In Matthew 17 it says the truth is if you have the faith as small as a mustard seed, you can say to this mountain, move from here to there and it will do it. Nothing is impossible.

Aside from praying, I would like to be kept in the loop of a normal life. I would love to have lots of mail of encouragement, inspiring, funny and everyday life. Tell us if you saw a good movie. We may be renting a few. Talk to us about real things and insignificant things, I'm sure we'll need it. We are setting up spokespeople to help us coordinate the things that we may need so that if you want news on me or to offer assistance, they could help you.

I am smiling right now. I have a great family and we're going to fight. We are not asking, why me? Rather, we are saying, try me! We can do this, please help lift us up. God's will be done, a lot of people are going to come out of our trials with a stronger faith, us included.

God Bless You,

Heather & Larry

And so it began. My letter and the news spread as planned. It was a great way for me to communicate. I could be direct without being worried about reactions from others. The spokesperson idea worked well from the start. Marnie was willing and able to dispense information for my coworkers. My brother Troy took on close friends and immediate family. Larry was able to handle the people he worked with. It helped people to feel involved and be able to provide support without it being a strain on me. Before long I would be reaping the benefits of this letter. Those that had been standing off moved in closer and a team began to form.

Snapshot: Colleen, Heather's Mother

"My initial reaction was simply shock. She was too young to get breast cancer. How could it be stage IV already? It should have been me. I would gladly change places.

"I took Heather to a bookstore right away looking for encouraging books, any information. We both love to read. However, I couldn't find anything encouraging past stage II. I bought everything that could give us some direction as to things we could do: medical treatment, alternative treatments, nutrition, etc. One week later when we found out it was stage IV and I heard about the doctor's reluctance to even try treatment, I vowed Heather would never see him again. I lit a fire under her brother Troy to find a doctor who would be positive and give her the best chance. He found Dr. Merajver at U of M, the most positive doctor we could have hoped for."

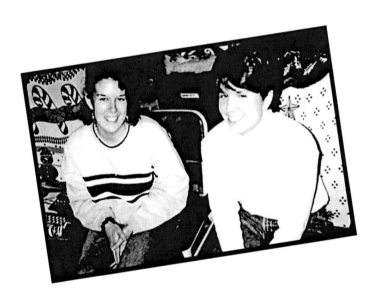

CHAPTER 6

Beginnings and Endings

Sydney Bs,

My job is to protect you, to care for you, to help you grow up. And then I'm diagnosed and I'm not sure that I can do that. Something you could never understand is going to impact every part of your life. That isn't fair to you, but life certainly isn't about fair.

We are each going to be better and stronger in the end. For now, though, please understand that mommy isn't going to be feeling very well all of the time, and that playing may not be a priority. You'll probably be with Daddy, Nana, and Grandma more than with me for a while, but we'll make it, and we'll savor every moment that we can.

God is with us. The doctors prayed with me after being diagnosed, seeking healing and restoration for my body. It is time to expect a miracle.

Love you,

Mommy

HAVING COMPLETED MY first chemo treatment and started the process of letting others know what was going on, I took my first steps toward surviving. In a matter of days I was bolstering my strength, being presented with resources, and dealing with the emotions that others and I were feeling. The last two weeks of December, Christmas vacation, was a difficult time in many ways as I tried to sort out my new challenges.

Since childhood, I had spent the two weeks around Christmas at our family timeshare in Sarasota Sands, Florida. It had always been the best two weeks of every year with family and friends. The tradition had begun with my parents, who had married just before Christmas and honeymooned half a mile from the family condo. Larry and I had continued the tradition, but this year was different.

Our families were profoundly sad, as we expected them to be. My mom and dad were around our house some and we were at theirs as well. We went through the motions of normal, but with a heaviness hanging over everything. I was in pretty regular communication with Troy as he would reassure me from afar that we were doing the right thing. However, I only spoke to Josh right after he had found out. He did his best to keep it normal, but honestly, he was a 19-year-old college freshman at the time. Like many other baby brothers, he was not usually in the position of comforting me.

In some ways it might have been even harder on Larry's family as they watched their son and brother stand by me knowing that he could be facing a world of hurt. We didn't spend as much time with them, but we knew they would do anything we asked. Thank God for Sydney. She brought light to every situation and gave us all something to focus on.

To escape the emotional pain I did my best to move forward and try to find things that I could do to make a difference. Meredith, my family doctor, had given me the name and phone number of her aunt, a doctor who was a breast cancer survivor in California. Meredith told me she had made a lot of changes in her diet and believed it had really made a difference. I called her one evening from my parents' house. Armed with a pen and legal pad I began to learn of things I could do to kill cancer. By the time I hung up I had a pad full of scribbles indicating I needed to dramatically change the way I ate. It was a bit overwhelming. She talked about meat, dairy, sugar, and white flour all being things that feed cancer as opposed to vegetables, fruits and whole grains which had the potential to reverse the disease process. I knew that I had a lot of work and research to do, but I was so grateful to have something I could control and participate in.

My mom immediately offered to do research. She has always been good at that kind of thing. Mom's friend Debbie had told her it was important that someone other than the patient do the research, as you have to schlep through a lot of dismal information to get to the good stuff. Debbie had been doing this research task for her son's very difficult battle with leukemia—and he had pulled through. The good information on LISTSERV and on websites can be lifesaving, but it is a treacherous place for a patient to be because of all of the emotional ups and downs that are out there. Yet, it is a positive when the medical community knows you are participating fully and are completely involved by doing your homework.

The upside to Christmas break was that I was doing well physically after my first chemo treatment. The medications I had been given as I left the hospital addressed virtually every problem I was encountering from an upset stomach to a head full of thoughts that wouldn't slow down making it almost impossible to sleep. My prayer journal describes it a bit better.

> *Dear Lord,*
> *This is a journey, a new one that I never expected. Cancer, not just a little bit, metastatic breast cancer, cancer in my bones. I feel healthy; I guess I'm not. I've had my diagnosis for 2 weeks now. Is it sinking in? I'm not sure, but it is always there. Last*

night I tried to sleep without drugs since chemo. It was not very restful, but I made it. Thank you for no strange racing thoughts. They are so bothersome. I'm not sure how to feel Lord. I trust you, I know how to fight. Do I just go on? Am I supposed to be reflecting on all of this and making something good happen? I don't know. Thank you for my life. I have a beautiful daughter that screeches and smiles for everyone. Help me to stay close to her, for her to want her mommy even if she is sick. Thank you for a husband whose commitment is stronger than I know. Please strengthen him. Thank you for a mom who is willing to have us all stay for as long as we need to. Lord, help me to focus on today—it doesn't seem so big then.

One night during the holiday break we went to the neighborhood Christmas party on the street where I grew up. It was a small gathering, mainly two other families that I had known all my life. I wasn't keeping in touch the same way they had, so I had lost that comfortable feeling of just hanging out. Add that to my cancer and everyone was uncomfortable. Thank God for kids. They always provide entertainment and something to talk about.

My closest friend growing up was there that night. Christy and I had racked up many hours as children doing all sorts of things from playing with dolls, to riding our dirt bikes, to swimming in the pool. In high school we hung with a large group of friends of which we were the center. Christy, two years my senior, let me drive long before anyone else, and provided me with my first college experiences. We had both gotten married within a year of each other and moved in different directions. Since that time, the phone calls had dwindled to a couple of times per year.

At the party, when Christy told me that she had just quit her job and would be able to do anything I needed, I didn't believe her. I had been hearing well-meaning offers for a couple of weeks already from all sorts of people. It was just what many people seem to say when they hear something tragic. I just nodded and said OK and went on with the night feeling empty, hollow and on the verge of desperate. What had happened to normalcy?

We spent Christmas Day with Larry's family at his parents' house. I did my best to enjoy it, but I really couldn't. Syd had fun, though. I honestly don't remember much more about the holidays that year except for the fact that our family was in different places. My mom and dad had made plans to go to Texas to visit family since we were not doing the annual trip to Sarasota Sands. With all that was going on, I asked my mom to stay home, which she did. My dad went with my brother Josh and our grandparents. They visited with family and spent a lot of time praying in Brownsville, Texas. At home, we looked for information that could help us and struggled to go on.

I continued to search for hope. One day my mom and I went to the Christian bookstore to find anything on the subject. She, in her grief, had said she would buy me any book I wanted. Normally, that would be a dangerous statement, as one of my favorite things to do is read. However, the selection was not great. Though I could find many books about cancer, they were so discouraging I couldn't read them. The one book I found to be helpful was *Chicken Soup for the Surviving Soul*. It spoke about conquering a lot of things—and conquering was something I wanted to know more about.

I bought a red spiral bound notebook to use as a journal of some sort. I picked red because it is bold and feisty. It has always been my favorite color. On the front cover I listed my name and address in case I left it somewhere. Under that I put a column for answered prayers. I wanted to be able to remind myself of God's hand in this. I began by listing U of M and Dr. Merajver. This notebook became my constant companion.

Mom and I also shopped for a wig. I wasn't sure I would ever wear it, but I wanted the option. I wanted to buy one before my hair came out, so they would know what I was supposed to look like. The older ladies in the shop were nice, though a little too sweet for me. We left with a wig. I was just glad it was done. It all seemed as artificial as the hair I had just purchased. It was as if we were out shopping for something I really wanted. Once again I was feeling sorry for myself, asking why I should have to be the one going through any of this.

As the Christmas season ended I faced my first day on my new job. I knew I wouldn't be working while doing chemo; I had too many other things to work on. I waited anxiously to go back on the Monday after the new year and then, because of bad weather, school was canceled. This wouldn't have been a problem except for the fact that Kelly had said that my hair would fall out in two weeks, which was Monday, and she was right on the money. I could reach up and pull just a little and out it came. I resisted because I wanted to look OK for my first day.

I went to work on Tuesday, spending the first minutes explaining to Human Resources that I needed to work one day to continue insurance benefits from my previous district to this one. They agreed without a problem. They would ask the board for a leave through the end of the school year. Being a brand new employee, the leave would likely be granted; but if I couldn't return by September, my job would likely be gone. It was a hard, hard day.

For the one full day I needed to work, I was placed in a pre-school classroom, basically as a classroom aide. People, who knew I was not an aide and had no idea why I was there, greeted me with a lot of puzzlement. I made small talk with people I had never met before, trying to avoid the whole issue of cancer that would only make me cry. As I drove home, I tugged at the hair on my head, pulling out handfuls of my thick, dark brown hair.

I was so glad to walk in the door. I wasn't a normal person anymore; I couldn't do normal things as if there wasn't cancer. When Larry got home, I told him I couldn't watch my hair fall out. Larry saw this as an opportunity and went for it. Sydney, Larry and I all crammed into the bathroom and went to work on it. It was quite an experience. We tried scissors, with Larry claiming he'd cut hair while in the Marines, and then it was clippers, and finally a razor to shave my head smooth. My husband can find the humor in anything. By the time we were done we were laughing so hard Sydney was staring at us, dumbstruck. He told me I looked great, making me feel much better. The shocking thing was it didn't look that bad to me either. The dread of no hair had been worse than the reality.

With my hair shaved off and an evening ahead of us, Larry suggested that we go out. We went to the basketball game at the high school where he taught. I would never have moved so quickly to go out into public, but with his encouragement I decided to do it. I would put this first time out behind me before I lost my nerve. So I found a bandana, put it on and off we went. I found I could do anything with him by my side.

The transformation was being made inwardly and outwardly. I began to realize that I had one focus right now: killing cancer. It was my essence—and the most important job in my life.

I never used the wig I purchased. It felt phony to me, an aid to be used to make other people comfortable. With a wig covering my baldness one might not even know that I had cancer and that was now the largest part of my life. I chose to deal with an occasional stare with the hope that people would accept me as I was. This was long before being bald was as accepted as it is now.

Snapshot: Christy, Heather's Best Friend

"I learned about the cancer from my mom. She called me. I can always tell when she doesn't want to tell me something. So, with hesitation, she proceeded to tell me that one of our neighbors heard in the teacher's lounge that Heather had breast cancer. I said, 'That can't be true' and I hung up on her. I don't think I had ever hung up on my mom before. She must have hung up the phone and cried, so my dad put on his coat and walked across the street to talk to Heather's parents to find out if it really was true.

"I don't remember very much right after that; there must have been a second phone call but I don't remember what was said. I do remember that I watched my wedding video so I could see her, and thinking: *She can't have breast cancer. It doesn't run in her family.* I found the book she gave me for my graduation from college and slept with it in my hands. The next day was a bit of a blur too. I went to work, but couldn't stop the tears from streaming down my face.

"My husband talked me into going to the mall after work since it was Christmastime 'to take my mind off of things.' All I remember was seeing a sea of faces, the sound of my own heart beating in my head, feeling the hot tears rolling down my cheeks and wanting to scream: *PLEASE SOMEBODY HELP MY FRIEND, SOMEBODY HAS TO BE ABLE TO HELP HER!!!*

"I knew I couldn't call and cry on her. I certainly wasn't going to make her comfort me. It took me a few more days to believe I was composed enough to call her. When I called, I got Heather's father-in-law. I just asked him to tell her that I called and tell her that I knew. She didn't have to tell me. I was thinking it was going to be really hard to tell her friends.

"I didn't know what to do or how to be helpful. All I knew for sure was that I wanted to help and that I could be there for her. Whatever happened I could be there. I didn't know anything about cancer. I didn't know the difference between chemo and radiation. I just thought I would want someone to be with me if I was scared."

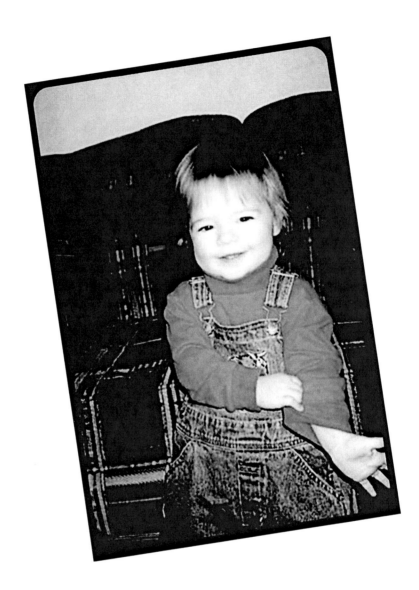

CHAPTER 7

Angels Among Us

Sydney Bs,

A fresh new day is a gift, though I never realized it before. Enjoying that day is our responsibility, a way of using the gift given to us. As a little one you are so good at enjoying things, delighted in a face that Daddy makes or throwing you up into the air. More words are coming out of your mouth every day; it is amazing. It is so good to be with you. I guess I need to thank the cancer for that, for being at home to see your smile. We are making it Hon; there are lots of people wanting to help us. Keep smiling.

Mommy

WITH THE NEW year starting we began a new routine. One moment I would be sure I was killing cancer and then a little ache would make me unsure of myself again. My husband, the coach, would step in and encourage me to keep moving forward. I don't know how I would have made it without his daily encouragement. I always think about the line from the movie *Dumb and Dumber* where the main character asks the woman about his chances of being her boyfriend. When she replies "one in a million" he responds with: "So you're telling me I have a chance!" I had decided that all I needed was a chance. Someone had to be the one in a million after all, why shouldn't it be me?

Whether or not I always believed it, I was making progress. The tumor was responding to the chemo and it was shrinking. I was feeling pretty good, though that dipped a bit with chemo. I laid low for a couple of days after getting it, but I was never actually sick.

After a couple of rounds of chemo, I added another doctor to my team. From the very beginning Dr. Merajver had spoken of doing a stem cell transplant. She referred me to Dr. Lois Ayash, part of the U of M Bone Marrow Transplant team. For all of Dr. Merajver's exuberance, Dr. Ayash was very reserved. Where Dr. Merajver consistently offered words of encouragement, Dr. Ayash spoke words of caution.

Dr. Ayash and I met on a chemo day in an exam room down the hall from Dr. Merajver. My mom and Larry were with me as usual. We had been told the stem cell procedure was pretty involved and Dr. Ayash said that we were welcome to record the conversation.

The meeting was fairly one-sided. Dr. Ayash laid out the procedure, the potential problems and the statistics for success. Transplants were clinical trials; there were lots of unknowns. More testing would be needed to determine whether or not I would even be a candidate.

I found myself really liking Dr. Ayash and having confidence in her. I wanted her to believe in me also, and made it a goal to be one of her "good statistics." When I told her as much, I got a small smile in return, spurring me forward.

I found out that after my last chemo session I would be doing a bone marrow biopsy to determine if there was cancer in my bone marrow. This was big. If there was no cancer, we would be able to proceed with a stem cell transplant in Ann Arbor. If there were still cancer cells present we would need to go to one of a few centers in the country where they can separate the cancer cells out before giving my stem cells back to me.

This whole process would allow the doctors to give me very high levels of chemo to stop the cancer and then give me life by reintroducing the cells I needed to fight infection.

Once at home, I added Dr. Ayash to my answered prayer column in my red notebook. I also added the extended leave that was granted from my new employer. I proceeded to write my second letter, which went out to a larger group than the first. I was getting encouragement from old friends and as well as new ones.

With things heading in the right direction from a medical standpoint, I needed to focus on life at home, which was still up and down emotionally. Over time, I found people that could step in and help me with my quest to regain my health. I realized later that these were the angels among us.

One early angel was Joanie, the mother-in-law of a teacher at one of the schools I had worked in. Joanie was a survivor of a similar diagnosis who had really done her homework. She had a wealth of information, which she shared wholeheartedly when I called her. She was very direct, telling me that I must make changes in my diet, get my mind fighting cancer, and pray. She was the first one to say with confidence, "You can do this. I will pray for you, you will pray for me, and we will both be OK." Joanie had been through hell. In the midst of her treatment she woke up one morning to find her husband had died in his sleep. She fought on with a determination that was clearly evident. Joanie traveled far and wide to find food that was good for her body, and she continually researched vitamins.

She treated fighting cancer like a job, and was telling me that I must do the same. I was touched that a woman who didn't even know me was so willing to help me. She invested a lot of time and energy encouraging me to take charge of my fight. She sent me recorded meditations to listen to every day to kill the cancer. They were created by Bernie Siegel, a medical doctor who fully believes in the mind-body connection. He has produced a lot of great material to help cancer patients utilize the power within themselves to heal. It was an amazing and powerful message.

My childhood friend Christy called back. It wasn't just to chat. She was asking what she could do and when would be a good time for her to visit. She had told her husband that this was a priority in her life, and she would be doing whatever she could for me. A few days later she drove the two and a half hours as if I was still just down the street. The friendship that was so much a part of my childhood blossomed again.

At church, my pastor he told me that God had good things in store for me. Pastor Noggle was not one to just say something for the sake of making conversation. I took this as another angel moment. So I began to believe this too.

Our neighbors, Mike and Beth Simon, were a constant source of help and support to us. We attended the same church and, truthfully, they were a big reason why we chose to go there. Mike and Beth really cared about us and they treated us like family, which was great considering our families were hours away. They, like us, did not have any extraordinary knowledge of cancer, but their desire to help in any way was obvious from the beginning. From helping with Syd, to making food, to having another place to go that felt comfortable—Mike and Beth provided it all.

We began to meet regularly to pray. Others would come as well, but Mike and Beth were a constant. We would get together at my house. Sometimes I would use my notebook to start us off and then we would each take a turn praying for specific things in my treatment, for my family, and for healing. It was a very powerful time—good for all involved, I believe. I learned to ask God and people for specific needs.

I discovered that the schools that I had worked in were full of angels. A large planter arrived from the Sheridan Elementary staff right after my diagnosis. Books and cards and little pick-me-ups came on a regular basis. Lakeview Elementary provided a lifeline of pizza gift certificates so my husband could eat regardless of my choice of dinner options for the night.

The teachers at my husband's school were amazing, offering all kinds of support. There were offers of sick days and financial help if needed. The support made school a great place for Larry to be. He could go there and focus on things other than cancer. Their kindness extended to me. I learned that cancer loves inactivity so I began to walk. The teachers offered to walk the halls with me. I would put Sydney in her stroller or I'd leave her with Larry and off we would go.

My family offered different types of reassurance. My brother Troy would tell me that the doctors were doing their very best. I began to call him each time something new was coming just to hear him tell me that he believed in it and that I could do it. It was a doctor's perspective with a dose of big-brother wisdom—a winning combination. Mom would tell me we would do whatever we needed to do. Every day we talked. Sometimes about big things, other times not. My younger brother, Josh, would say he believed in me. My dad would tell me that he loved me.

Larry's family wanted to help out in any way possible. Larry's mom and his sister Kathy became Sydney's regular babysitters for all of our visits to Ann Arbor. Larry's sister Kim sent me a package from Minnesota where she lived. Included in it was a tabletop stone fountain whose trickling water sounded so peaceful. It was healing.

I'm not exactly sure how Pam came in to my life. She also taught school and attended our church, but I never knew her well. Her husband, Jim, had died of cancer a few years before I was diagnosed. He was a teacher at the high school, a coach, loved by many. Pam was left with two school-aged children to raise on her own. Pam also believed in nutrition, positive thinking and prayer. She offered me all sorts of resources in our very small community. Her radiant spirit calmed me. She joined my group of those who believed in my ability to kill cancer. She told me that we would do anything we needed to, hire a chef, go see different doctors, whatever it took. Pam believed that Jim could have survived if he had had the strength to fight by using diet, exercise and meditation. Pam always had encouraging words for me, words that had substance that led me forward in my fight.

One day I was feeling a little lost and a blue Toyota minivan pulled up to my house. Out of the van came Chris, with a small book and a chubby, ceramic angel holding scripture. Chris grew up in the same small town that my husband did and now lived close by. She was a kindergarten teacher, with an easy smile and long, straight brown hair, often drawn back in a loose bun. It is hard not to be cheered when in a conversation with her. The book that she brought was entitled, *Healed of Cancer*, by Dodie Osteen. A friend who had dealt with cancer had recommended it to her. Chris wanted to help, and this is what she was led to do. The book had a profound effect on my thoughts, providing a spiritual basis to fight the cancer. It made me want to stand up and cheer. I read it constantly, wrote down all the verses in my red notebook. This notebook that I purchased in my darkest days was becoming my greatest source of hope. I filled it with everything that encouraged me.

My husband, Larry, was incredible. He was always there to believe in me; he backed me in everything I did. As a coach, he is a great encourager and calm in a crisis. He would listen to me when I was scared and reassure me at every turn. Above all, he treated me like I was normal. He found the humor in everything. He honored the best parts of our relationship prior to cancer and had the grace to accept the changes as well. That was the best thing he could have done.

Whenever I was wondering if I was on the right track, God jumped in with reassurance or another angel. One time it was sent by Kathy, my husband's aunt. Kathy has this personality that draws people to her, a ray of sunshine on the darkest of days. She lived in Ann Arbor. She made it a point to connect me with Diana Dyer. Diana is a registered dietitian and three-time cancer survivor. She had thoroughly researched food and supplements to impact her fight. Out of the experience she wrote a great resource, *A Dietitian's Cancer Story*. It was packed with all types of information, menus, shopping lists and, my favorite, a shake recipe. The shake included soy, veggies, fruit and lots of other good stuff. I took to it immediately. I found it was a great way to start my day.

The other book that Kathy sent along was by Greg Anderson, a 15-year survivor of the 30-days-to-live diagnosis. His book was called *50 Essential Things To Do When The Doctor Says It's Cancer*. It was great for me. It laid out the plan that I was pursuing: good conventional medicine, time with God, exercise, nutrition and a purpose in life. He spoke of the healing notebooks he had filled on his journey. I drank it in. Every few chapters it would say to take a break and I would be bummed. I wanted to consume it all.

Greg Anderson had started a group called the Cancer Conquerors (now the Cancer Recovery Foundation of America) and in the back of the book it told how you could become a member. I had grown to dislike the wishy-washy "do what you can" approach and was very interested in being a conqueror. The word resonated throughout my body. I joined right away. I was all for aligning myself with people who were taking cancer head-on; those who were not afraid to say, "I will fight."

On the angel front, I had someone to watch Sydney every day so I could spend some intense time fighting cancer through prayer, exercise and meditation. Lois, Sydney's adopted grandma, had been watching her most of her life. She continued to watch Syd, and refused to be paid. I had offers for meals every day, most of which I declined because of the changes I was making in my diet.

My days began to settle into a pattern. I would get up in the morning and take Sydney to Lois' and then return home. At home, I would make a shake while listening to a *Songs for Life* CD. I would go for a walk, listening to my music, knowing that God was in control, but wanting Him to want me to win this battle. There was a song on the CD, "Warrior is a Child" by Twila Paris, that hit me hard. It speaks of appearing to be strong, winning battles left and right, but in reality being just a child, scared and at times, tired. The many hours spent walking on my snow-covered dirt road were so good for me. They revived my body and my mind. I would come in and make a cup of hot green tea, read through all of my healing verses, and then lie down and listen to Bernie. Together we would target the cancer and make that area strong again. After that, I could then make a nutritious lunch and go to get my daughter.

There was a period initially when I struggled with sending Sydney away while I was at home. My outlook began to shift though, and I began to think of this time as an investment in our future. If Sydney had been home I could have made her breakfast and taken her on my walk. The focus would have been different. It would have been on her needs rather than my own. The more I read, the more I realized that I needed to take care of myself, and do it well. It wasn't selfish. It was necessary. By spending time alone each day I could give the rest of my day to my family, without guilt or regrets.

Snapshot: Mike and Beth, Neighbors and Friends

"Our most enduring and endearing memory of Heather's battle with cancer is the day she and Larry informed our Sunday Bible Study Group of her diagnosis. She was, of course, emotional as she shared the news with us. Her concern, however, was not with the cancer so much as it was with whether God's presence would remain with them during this difficult time in their lives. Even in the shadow of this diagnosis she was determined to have her faith in God—that His power be the defining aspect of her battle with the disease. We are impressed by her desire to have God and His love shine through her. Her statement, often repeated throughout the years that followed: 'I want people to see God at work in my life helping me fight cancer,' is still an inspiration to us when we encounter difficult times.

"I told Heather that I had made a decision early on to help in any way I could," Beth continued. "She remembers me telling her that though I was unsure of what the outcome might be, if she was going to be pulling as hard as she was on the oars of the boat, I certainly was not going to be the anchor."

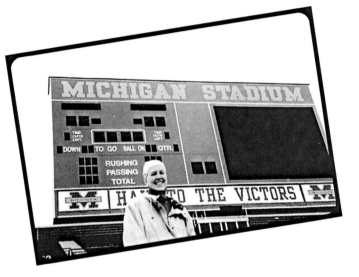

CHAPTER 8

The Rest of the Puzzle

Sydney Bs,
You can do anything that you want to do. It probably won't be easy, but you can do it. Don't live in fear of failure. Stand up and plow through to get to your goal. I think we limit ourselves so much sometimes, because we don't think we can. You don't limit yourself right now. It doesn't matter if you fall down, you will get back up and try again to reach the goal. And if you fall again, you'll get up again, knowing that the goal is worth the struggle. What a great quality. It seems a shame that we teach it away.

The words keep coming, and some of them break my heart. The other day you found an empty bottle that you held up with a question forming. "Mommy medicine?" you asked. Yes, Mommy's medicine, I wish you didn't have to know. I love you.

Mommy

THE DAY CAME for my bone marrow biopsy. Dr. Ayash was doing the procedure and she told me it would be a bit uncomfortable as I didn't have a lot of cushion on my tush. Uncomfortable was an understatement. She used a long needle to extract marrow from my pelvic bone on each side. It is quite an experience to have someone leaning into you with all her strength. I was glad when it was over.

As I got up I said, "It's going to come back clean."

Dr. Ayash, with a little smile, shook her head as if to say I hope so.

With many aspects of my treatment rolling along, chemo every third Monday, prayer meetings, regular exercise and meditation, I found myself struggling with what exactly I should be eating. I knew nutrition was very important, but the amount of information was staggering. It ranged from a strict macrobiotic diet to eating whatever you want because you need the calories.

Having spoken with Meredith's aunt and later with Joanie, I had the idea that a vegetarian lifestyle might be permanent. Reading Diana's book confirmed that thought, with the exception of fish. I did not have a problem with this, but I wanted a concrete plan. I made an appointment with the dietitian at the U of M Cancer Center and had great expectations. It didn't work out as I had hoped. The dietitian was very nice and knowledgeable, but not ready to move as quickly as I wanted. I left with a transitional diet to vegetarianism—but I was already past that step.

My mom, having gone to the appointment with me, told me about Block Medical Center in Evanston, Illinois. She suggested calling them.

She said, "Evanston isn't that far away. If it's going to help it doesn't matter where it is. Just call and see what they say. Keith Block's name has come up in three books that I have read. I think it's worth checking it out." My mom, the researcher, strikes again.

A couple of days later I called. It was so easy. I explained my situation and that I would like to talk to someone about my diet.

The woman on the phone asked me to send my medical records. They would set me up with a doctor, and then I would see the nutritionist. We made the appointment for my husband's birthday, February 15.

Larry, my mom and my dad all went with me to Block. We drove down the night before and had dinner at a great Mexican restaurant a block behind the Block Center. The day of my visit we all showed up and a nurse drew my blood. I hadn't been allowed to eat that morning because of the blood work. Being accustomed to a large breakfast I was starved, so after the draw we were shown into an unusual examining room where they brought me a healthy snack. The room had an examining table, the usual blood pressure equipment, and a loveseat like you would find at home—big, soft, and luxurious. Instead of paper gowns, there were cloth ones and real throw blankets. There was also a beautiful view of Lake Michigan.

After being in so many places to do tests or see doctors, this room was a beautiful respite. It was a place where you were a person, not just a patient. The comfort of the real blanket and cloth gown spoke of quality and care in this throw-away world. Having real furniture rather than three vinyl covered chairs made the room inviting, a place to settle in and talk.

The snack threw me, too. I felt as though I was eating someone's lunch. There were organic raisins, a box of organic apple juice, a sort of windmill cookie and nondairy butterscotch pudding. I had gotten my green tea when we came in because it was offered instead of coffee. I knew that I was in for something different.

Having already met the nurse, she reviewed the past months of my life and performed the usual basic exam. Dr. Kut came in shortly after. She was not the picture that I have for a doctor. She was beautiful, stylishly dressed, with dark flowing hair that was far more than just combed quickly that morning. She didn't wear a lab coat, eliminating another barrier between doctor and patient.

Dr. Kut went through my history, asking questions about my current treatment and plans for the future. She questioned certain drugs, and agreed with the current protocol. She explained that she would be happy to offer a second opinion in my situation, since she also often prescribed chemotherapy for her patients. I really liked her. I felt she was honest, unobtrusive and very knowledgeable. She was clearly able to handle my treatment.

After Dr. Kut left I dressed then my family gathered in the room for the nutritionist. Where Dr. Kut was a slim person with a soft voice, David Grotto filled the room with his presence. He stood over six feet; and though not overweight, there was a bigness about him, gusto if you will.

"Heather, I'm David Grotto, so nice to meet you."

After introducing my family and exchanging pleasantries about the trip, we began to delve into nutrition. David provided a wealth of information, much of which was laid out in a three ring binder. He told us about Dr. Block, the founder of the center, and the research he continually does to make sure that what goes into our bodies is beneficial. David went on to talk about how amazing the human body is. It has the ability to fight all sorts of diseases, but it needs the proper nutrients. The goal is to make the immune system as strong as possible, to get as much benefit as possible from the conventional treatment that I would be receiving, and to eliminate foods that feed cancer.

We began to talk about foods to eliminate. This list included many things I had grown up eating. Meat and dairy products were gone. My cancer was hormone-receptive and I did not need the hormones that come naturally or synthetically through the shots that are given to livestock to increase production. Meat and dairy also have unnecessary antibiotic content and a lot of fat. When I asked about calcium, David told me about other great ways to get calcium. Hydrogenated and partially hydrogenated oils were next on the list of things to go, followed by sugar and all of its family members.

I began to wonder what was left when David began to talk about what he would like to see me eat each day: Vegetables—especially dark green leafy, cruciferous, and root; fruit—highlighting berries; whole grains—brown rice, whole wheat breads, whole grain noodles; for protein—beans, some fish and soy products. By the time it was listed out, I knew it would be a challenge to eat it all. I asked David about my shake from Diana's book. He had just had her on the radio show that he hosted talking about her book and her plan. I was shocked to find that he knew her, and that he could put a stamp of approval on my shake with no trouble.

Along with dietary needs, David also addressed the area of supplements. I had gotten advice from many people at this point as to what type of vitamins I should be taking. I was left wondering how much of anything I should take as well as what brand I should be using. Were more expensive vitamins better? I had no idea. David told me how at Block they would use blood tests to determine and monitor the function of my immune system and my vitamin levels. From there they would prescribe supplements to optimize these. I was able to buy supplements from Block, feeling confident that they were of great quality because of the research that was ongoing. This was a huge relief to me to be able to let someone else do the work and get supplements specific to my needs.

I left Evanston armed with a way to starve cancer and build a strong immune system. More important, I left with validation that I could make a difference in this fight. I couldn't wait to get started.

Once home, I began my new way of eating, feeling confident that I had the rest of the puzzle. I live in a small farming community, where vegetarians are nonexistent, for the most part. However, God once again opened doors. My vitamins were shipped right to my front door. Pam, my new friend, introduced me to the co-op she belonged to. I could order once a month and pick up my food at a local elementary school. Then, the consignment shop in town closed, only to be replaced by

Hometown Health Foods. I couldn't believe it. Even Helen's, the local restaurant, began to serve veggie burgers on whole wheat buns with bottled water.

Snapshot: David Grotto, Heather's Dietitian

"Heather and I met when I was working at the Block Center. I remember that Heather had a lot of people with her. Another thing that stuck with me was that unlike many people who tend to be outwardly anxious, she seemed to have control. This was helpful in that she showed a strong desire to learn about what to do and how she could partner in the battle. At that meeting I shared some research that had just come out stating that those who were engaged in their own care did better in terms of survival. I could see that Heather was ready to do just that. She and her family asked good questions and seemed ready to apply all she was learning.

"Over time, it has been enjoyable to watch as Heather used her circumstances as an opportunity to help others. To take the information and turn that in to a mission has been a good thing. People have benefitted from Heather sharing her success.

"One of the things that I tell people with cancer is to try to take a lifelong approach to it. I think it helps to think about how best to control cancer. Heather has lived that way for quite some time now. It also makes sense to use a disease like cancer to kick up your overall health and view it as a lifelong commitment to a healthier lifestyle."

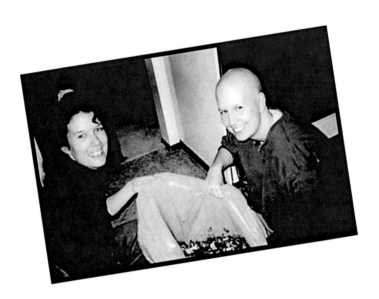

CHAPTER 9

Preparing

Sydney Bs,
What is it that I really want you to know? Let's see: That I love you and I still can't believe that you are mine. That no matter what happens, I am fighting as hard as I can to watch you grow up. That God has a plan in all of this. Some days I still can't believe that I really have cancer, although if I didn't, we certainly would be going through a lot of unnecessary stuff. I still feel guilty for leaving you to work on me, but I'm praying it will be worth it. It's amazing how easily you adapt. Hair or no hair I'm still Mommy. You're the best.
Love you,
Mommy

WHEN I WAS first diagnosed with cancer, every single test revealed more cancer, more problems and bleaker outcomes. As we moved along, we were getting better news, which I decided to share with my supporters.

Dear Friends,

The Psalms tell us to let everything that has breath praise the Lord. We are praising, and singing, and high-fiving every day. We are killing cancer!! In the past five days my doctor has told me that she could no longer measure the 5-centimeter mass in my breast; and the bone marrow biopsy that we asked you to pray for came back clean, without cancer. My brain scan also came back clean a few weeks ago. God is hearing our prayers, and we, again, want to thank you for your faithfulness. Aside from the medical stuff, I feel great. I have lots of energy. On a daily basis, I've been working out, trying to eat 9–11 fruits and veggies, drinking tons of water, taking vitamins and spending quiet time with God. If you are a "what's next" person, this is the scoop. I've finished my normal chemo. Next I'll begin stem cell collection so that they can freeze them and give them back later. This should take 2–4 days. My hospital admission date is March 17. At that time I'll begin 96 hours of continuous chemo with the goal of killing all lurking cancer cells. I'll then get my stem cells back. When my counts are high enough that I can fight some infection, they'll let me out. The plan is that I would repeat another intensive chemo session in 6–8 weeks with another stem cell transplant at that time. Please pray that my insurance company approves this repeat procedure. They have done that in the past, but currently have denied it for me.

I have a job for anyone who reads this letter and keeps us in their thoughts and prayers. I'm aware that there are far more of you than I know, so I am asking that you send me a picture. If you would like to send your favorite verse or quote I would appreciate that also. I have a healing notebook, which I want to fill with inspiration. The pictures will be a source of entertainment for me when I am in the hospital. Not because I expect them to be funny-looking, rather because I plan on putting them in my photo album during my three-week hospital stay. I'm a visual person and would really appreciate having a face connected with all the good thoughts that I've gotten from each of you. Peace to all.

Heather

We began to get good news from my test results. The way Dr. Merajver delivered them made it even better. After my brain scan came back normal, she said nonchalantly, "I knew you were thinking all right."

As for the breast tumor being undetectable, she told me, "We are clobbering the cancer!" I loved her enthusiasm and her confidence. It energizes me to this day.

Having also made good on my statement to Dr. Ayash that my bone marrow biopsy would be clear, I was well on my way to a stem cell transplant. My doctors wanted to do one more round of testing to see where we were at in terms of progression of disease.

By this time I knew each test or scan and could help others understand what each one entailed. There was the bone scan, which I called the tanner because of the way it closed down on top of you. The CT scan, or the lifesaver, because you passed through the middle of a round hole. And there was my least favorite, the MRI, which I deemed the thermos, the one you went into headfirst.

Around the time that I was preparing for the stem cell transplants I was reading a book called, *A Year of Miracles*. It is about an Ann Arbor woman who used a lot of meditative techniques. She worked with a doctor to make individualized meditations for each aspect of her treatment. Since I had had such good results by calling Block Medical Center, I decided to call this doctor, too. I got an appointment arranged so that I could have recorded meditations ready in time for my stem cell transplant. Together, in the course of three or four sessions, we were able to put together a meditative sequence specific to the drugs I would be using.

The stem cell collection took two days. Of all the procedures I had done to this point, this was my least favorite. In order to collect stem cells, a large needle is inserted in the crux of each arm. The blood goes out through one needle and circulates through a machine that is able to collect stem cells before the blood goes back into your body through another needle in the other arm. The procedure took about three hours to go through all the blood in the body. Although it did not hurt, I was unable to move my arms at all for the entire time. No itching my nose, no taking a drink, no changing the channel. Agony. I relied on my mom or Christy as I was stiff-armed, and they got me through it.

After finishing the stem cell collection the second day, Christy and I went to Whole Foods. We purchased the food we were using to prepare meals for the time I was in the hospital. I knew I would have a tough time following my diet while I was there so we decided to bring in food instead. We bought tons of produce, much of which we had never tasted before. We prepared lots of dishes, such as burritos, all of which could be easily frozen. Unfortunately, we found out later that none of them were very tasty. We learned the hard way that tasting along the way is crucial.

Christy was house sitting at her parent's house so we took all of our veggies back there. In many ways that night seemed as though we were back in high school again. We were hanging out together, just having fun. The radio was on, and the mood was light. We cleaned and mixed the massive amount of veggies. It got to be such a large quantity that no bowl was big enough to hold it all. We ended up shaking them up in a garbage bag in order to incorporate it all. At the end of the night, I called U of M and was ecstatic to learn that they had enough stem cells and I wouldn't need to go back for another day of torture.

With the stem cells collected and frozen, I could go home to begin gathering things to take back with me to the hospital. It was to be at least a three-week stay, so I was moving in. I put together a lot of pictures of Sydney and our family. I wanted everyone who came into my room to know that I was a real person with a real life, not a bald, sick creature who only existed in the hospital. I made a large sign that said, "Every day we are killing cancer." I was serious about that. I knew what I was there to do and I wanted everyone else on board. I brought all of my scrapbooking stuff, my meditative recordings and "Songs for Life" CDs.

In *A Year of Miracles,* that author talked about the healing quilts that she made. She had taken one with her each time to the hospital. I wanted to do the same.

Christy and I were going to make it together. When we finally got down to it we were under the gun, having started just two days before I was to be admitted. Christy came up on Sunday evening and we set up our sewing machines across the table from each other. Even though Christy's mom was known for making incredible quilts, Christy had no experience.

It was a great night. We sewed and sewed, ripped a few seams apart, and sewed some more. Late the next day we were finished, having spent a few hours crawling around on the floor to tie it together rather than quilting it. We had our moments of giggles, laughing at ourselves for the predicaments that we put ourselves in. The quilt looked amazing, with vibrant colors, beautiful florals, and of course U of M maize and blue.

I was prepared. I was ready to go.

Snapshot: Larry, Heather's Husband

"When we first got the diagnosis, it wasn't real. We got up the next day and it still wasn't real. We went to church and told some people but it still wasn't real. But every day it got a little more real. As more people found out, the diagnosis got more and more real. It went from holy crap to no big deal.

"As Heather shifted into I'm-going-to-kick-its-butt mode, I found myself shifting into coach mode. I knew how to be a coach. This was familiar ground when nothing else made sense. I had found my job. I was there to make her laugh, reassure, coach her on, reaffirm her when I wasn't so sure myself, encourage her, fix what was wrong. I used my ability to detach myself so I could make the next play in this game while trying to make everything as easy as it could be.

"The lowest point for me was when we found out. From then on, everything was good. How could it be worse? Every meeting, phone call, visit from a friend, appointment or interaction was good.

"We may have had it easier than some. Heather was young; we had wonderful friends, a great church, a terrific school community and strong families. The situation was not a natural thing for me at first. My initial reaction was not to ask for help. My attitude was that this is my problem and I should be able to handle it on my own. I think I learned a lot from this. People offered help and I learned to say yes. I learned how great people are.

"We did not want to impose on others and we said no too many times before we'd say yes. I was amazed by how willing others were to help and how much the little things can mean. A hand-written card, a phone call, an email, etc. I know what they can do.

"Through the cancer diagnosis, I learned there were people out there to help. I learned I didn't have to do it on my own. Cancer did not happen to me, it happened to Heather. But now I know if something bad did happen, I think I could handle it. We were pretty young when all of this happened. It was one heck of a lesson to learn. We had to grow up and learn some real life stuff. I grew up faster as a father and a husband.

"Cancer changed Heather; it changed me; and it changed our marriage. I know I hear about couples that are torn apart by cancer. I don't understand this. This challenge proved we were on the same team.

"The good that came of this was that Heather had to become a much more confident person. Her decision to fight this in spite of the awful odds was amazing. Our faith never felt as strong and as close as during all of this. This changed my faith forever. It was a commitment to trust God in a whole new way.

"I can remember the moment when the doctor told us before chemo that there were not going to be more kids. I did not know that. It was a surprise. Later, we decided to adopt. Family did not have to be by birth. I was OK with that. We joke with the kids today, 'We can always get more of you.'

"Most of the time things felt normal to me—it was not all 'cancer-time.' We would talk about the mundane daily things, we went to games, we went to church and we watched TV. These normal times helped me get through. I had to do the normal stuff for me if not for Heather.

"Somewhere along the line I had a conversation with God about Heather. I thanked Him for our miracle. I figured after this He was not going to change His mind and have the cancer come charging back—or at least I could not live my life believing that God would do this. It made no sense. This was my sort of coming-to-peace with the doctor visits since that initial year. We've had a couple of scares, but we've come through. I have to believe in this."

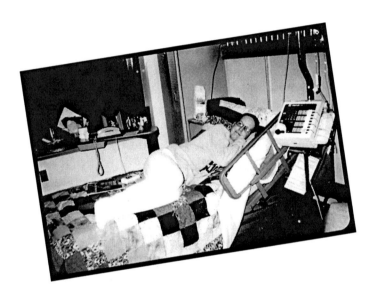

CHAPTER 10

The Spa

Sydney Bs,
I hate how different your life is from other little ones your age. Your parents talk about cancer, your mommy has to go away for a while. Will it affect you? Maybe make you stronger? I really don't know. I don't want you to be mad at God if I'm not always here. I think it would just be part of the plan, though we don't know why. You are going to be a great girl. You've got your daddy's rhythm, picking up a beat just like nothing. I wonder if you'll be in the band. Or maybe play a sport. Who knows? I'll be thinking of you Syd.
I love you,
Mommy

MY MARCH 17 admit date had arrived. Though I'm not Irish, I was hoping to borrow a little of their luck. The night before I left we gathered together to pray. It was a powerful time, circled together in our living room. Sydney walked around and played as though nothing was happening, but it surely was, we were crying out to God.

And so, Wednesday morning, with the car packed full of stuff, we went first to the Cancer Center. I couldn't believe I was stepping indoors for at least three weeks. I love being outside, even if just to walk to the mailbox.

Before being admitted I needed to have a central line placed in order to be hooked up to all the medicine. Up until this point whenever I got chemo or they needed blood I would get an IV. The line was necessary for a several reasons: I wouldn't be able to handle the amount of needle sticks that would be needed; some of the drugs the doctors were using were so powerful they wouldn't allow them to travel up my arm to enter my body; and there would often be more than one type of fluid entering my body at any given time.

I was given the option early on in my chemotherapy to have a port placed so that a nurse or the vampires could easily access my veins. I chose not to have this done as I didn't want something jutting out of my body to make me look different. I was already bald. My goal was to remain as human as possible in terms of equipment. It was a hang-up of mine, but I often felt that I was viewed as a disease, not a person, and the port seemed like one step closer to succumbing to the identity of a victim of cancer.

The line placement was treated rather casually, as the doctor who performed it does it all the time. It wasn't until later that it sunk in that the man had cut my jugular vein in order to place the tube that came out of my body near my collarbone. The tubing had an end on it where three syringes or lines could go. It looked like the wiring on a car that you connect the trailer lights to. Now that I could be "plugged in," I was ready to go upstairs.

Christy and I had been calling my room at the hospital "the spa". It seemed so much more appealing to check into a spa to do some intense healing. In reality it wasn't appealing at all, but instead, very sterile and uninviting. The University of Michigan Health System is immense, and just walking to my room, on floor 8A, from the Cancer Center involved a maze of hallways and elevators. After we found the correct wing I was shown to my room. The staff informed me that flowers had arrived for me before I had gotten there but since they were live I would not be able to enjoy them in my room. Already my show of support from friends had begun. After Larry made three very long trips to the car and back, I had all of my stuff and was ready to settle in.

I filled my windowsill with pictures of my family and me when I still had hair. I had a view of the helicopter pad so I could watch landings and take-offs. On the bulletin board went the sign that read, "Every day we are killing cancer," so that all could see it. I stashed my scrapbooking supplies, my puzzles and laptop and set up the card table that I had brought to work on. I left out the Magna Doodle and other small toys for Sydney to play with when she could visit. I filled the patient refrigerator with foods that I felt were good for me. I also had a basket of dried fruits and other snacks in my room. Into my top drawer went my healing notebook and Bible. Finally I spread my quilt on my bed, and the color snuffed the feeling of sterility. Be it ever so humble, it was nothing like home.

In came the nurses, raving over the quilt, getting ready to start the 96 hours of continuous chemo. I was ready with my meditative recordings when they were ready to start the first chemo drug.

And so it began, my time in the spa, with a nurse plugging in a line and letting the chemo flow while I listened to my visualizations and directed it to find any lurking cancer cells. I believed that my body was meant to kill cancer and that God had plans for my future. It was a serene and focused start to my stay.

Larry left that evening to go home. He was beginning three weeks of juggling work and taking care of Sydney, while his wife was in the hospital two and a half hours away. He took it all in stride. Larry, Christy and my mom had become a great support team for me and in some ways for each other. Because they could share the load it made it easier for all of us.

That night before I went to sleep I called Christy, "You are gonna be here tomorrow, right?"

"Yep. Want me to bring you a shake for breakfast?"

Ahhh, good friends. Where would I be without her? The more time that Christy and I spent together, the more our relationship solidified. We could laugh or cry, depending on what we needed. We had literally known each other from the day I was born. We were becoming closer than many sisters.

As the chemo flowed in I found myself feeling really good physically and emotionally. I got to work on a scrapbook full of inspiration and well-wishes that I had received; I perused all of the take-out menus that were brought to me by Aunt Kathy. She told me just to place my order and someone would bring it up. It was the book that Kathy gave me that introduced me to the shake. She and her husband, James, who is a chef, began to make and bring them each morning. My diet quickly put the hospital dietitian on the defensive. She was unable to keep track of calories consumed since I wasn't eating hospital food. She was also very concerned that the shakes would have something in them that would infect me. Needless to say, she and I had differing opinions about nutrition.

On Friday night the chemo started to knock out my immune system, and it hit me hard. I had Chinese for dinner, and having just consumed some great fried rice I found myself feeling ill. I threw up all of the rice, and it was the last thing that I ate for days. My counts were all beginning to drop and I felt terrible. The switch had been thrown and I was no longer in control. I had no energy. Everything that I put in my mouth I threw up. I would feel like I could do something and then decide it would be better just to lie on my bed. As the days went by the dietitian's aide stopped asking me to fill out a menu and instead just smiled warmly and put it on my table.

There were many mornings where it was difficult to stand long enough to get my weight without getting dizzy and needing to lie down. Though my job as an occupational therapist had people getting up and ready by themselves in the hospital, I thought the nurses were crazy when they made me take a shower every day. The last thing on my mind was a shower. I was concentrating on standing, or sometimes just sitting without feeling woozy. They, however, seemed to have all the confidence in the world, leaving me to stand on my own in hot water, telling me if I needed to I could sit down. That is what I call tough love.

Every morning Tracy, a PA, and the medical residents would round. Her visit was my way of gauging how I was really doing medically. I would try to read her expressions and comments to see if I was on par with where she expected me to be. During these visits Tracy would check my counts and adjust medications. She would also play on the Magna Doodle that was there for Sydney. Tracy loved that thing. After drawing a cat or some other doodle she would record my counts on a chart on my bulletin board.

No matter the day, I had a lot of visitors. Each day Larry, Christy or my mom came to be with me. A lot of days they all came. My room was where they met to pick up or deliver Sydney and to figure out how to get me the things I wanted or needed. My mom did all of the dirty work, such as my laundry and special requests. It was she who would be there if others couldn't, or she would take Sydney so Larry could be with me. Larry's sister came up one night, Meredith's parents stopped in, as well as her brother and others from the Christian Medical Association. Even the Cooking Girls from my church ventured down and Pastor Jim visited a few times. Mail continued to pour in, eight or nine cards a day as well as many emails racking up on my laptop. Oftentimes I was too tired to look at any of it.

Sydney was not a fan of my room. It was all too strange for her and she would hardly acknowledge me in that weird place. She preferred to ride the escalators. Though I understood, it was a bummer.

We watched as my white blood counts decreased each day and then bottomed out at 7, normal being in the range of 4,000-10,000. With my counts bottomed out and the life cycle of the chemo finished I was able to get my stem cells back. It was Wednesday, March 24. I had been in the hospital for one week. I was excited for the big day, thinking it would change the way I felt quickly. Larry was planning on being there for the big event, but he ended up with the flu. It was so bad that he was having trouble taking care of Syd. Christy drove up to our house to get Sydney and my mom came to the hospital to videotape the procedure.

My expectations for the stem cell transplant did not live up to the procedure. Tracy came in with a small bag, just like the ones that get hung on an IV pole. It just looked like frozen blood. She put it in a bowl of water to unthaw the cells and then began to put them in my line using a large syringe. I began to cough a dry, hacking cough, which she had said would happen because of the preservative. Slowly, she put the stem cells in and as she finished I threw up, also due to the preservative. That was it—a little cough, a little puke and then life. *Grow, grow, grow.*

I had thought I wasn't feeling well before the stem cells, and then I found out what not feeling well really felt like. My mouth and throat felt terrible, like the worst sore throat imaginable. The technical term was mucositis, and because of it I was started on a morphine drip. I was still unable to eat and I began to run fevers with unknown origins. During these days my visitors continued to visit though I didn't usually participate in anything related to them. Apparently, sometimes I did join in, but I have no recollection of the conversations. My mom, Larry or Christy were there just in case I would want to talk.

One day Christy's dad came up with her to see me. He was shocked at how easily Christy navigated her way first through the parking structure and then the maze of hallways and elevators in order to find me. Our lives had changed so much that she didn't even stop to think about being in this huge medical center as unusual.

I felt terrible and I was also really tired of being in the hospital. I was so weak I required help to get to do almost everything, including getting to the bathroom. That was fine during the day when my family was around. However, when I needed help at night it took forever for someone to come. When I would finally get back to sleep, in they'd come to wake me up. As the days wore on, I began to hate the aides who came in at 5:30 a.m. just to take my vitals. Every morning they made me get out of my nice warm bed to stand on the scale.

I realized something in the middle of one of my sleepless nights. I realized that no matter how much help I had fighting cancer, ultimately, it was just God and me. No one else would ever know exactly what it felt like to do what I was doing. As much support as I had, in the middle of those dark nights it was just Him and me. It made me realize how the life we live is only our own. It was me with God to lean on.

I did lean too. On one of those early mornings I found my chest feeling very heavy and breathing was not coming easily. My doctors ordered a chest X-ray and discovered that I had developed pneumonia. I had cancer, wasn't that enough? I didn't need any other problems. After all I had gone through I didn't want something like pneumonia to get the best of me. I knew the real risks of the transplant were more related to my immune system being weak and not being able to fight off things like pneumonia. Yet it made me really angry. It was another stumbling block to an already difficult time.

I can't imagine enduring a longer transplant, though I know many people do it. It was such a struggle internally to stay focused on healing or even some days, just to care. I could see the juggling that it took to manage my care as well as Sydney's too. It really took an army of people to get us through.

After having my transplant and enduring ten days of hell, my stem cells were up and growing. The morphine was discontinued and I began feeling better and started pushing like crazy to get out. Dr. Ayash had the patience of a saint as I bugged her on rounds every day. I went from this lifeless being to a supercharged, overconfident annoyance.

Toward the end of my stay, Christy and I spent hours talking. I've come to believe that there are very few people in the world that you are comfortable enough to be with for hours on end, no matter what the situation. We had a lifetime of memories to draw on though, and passed time rather easily. She would do laps with me, pushing my IV pole through the halls of 8A, or we would hang out in my room trying to figure out what was happening to our lives. The changes weren't all bad, but they were all-encompassing and deep. Christy had jumped into things with both feet, trying everything new thing that I did. It was awesome.

The day of my discharge we found ourselves having a discussion about how healthy we were. We were learning so much, how every day has so much to offer, how we spend far too much time on things that don't actually matter, and how we have a say in how our lives turn out. We were healthy, we were eating well, exercising and nurturing our spiritual lives. It was crazily ironic to think that my cancer made life more abundant than we had ever known.

Snapshot: Aunt Kathy, Larry's Aunt

"Heather's husband, Larry, was born when I was in college. I watched him grow up, graduate from high school, go off to the Marines, return to attend college and find Heather. It was a pretty good plot line that included the birth of what we all assumed was the first of many children, Sydney. Then the plot line went horribly wrong. It came in a phone call informing us that Heather was in trouble.

"I honestly don't remember much about the call other than it was bad. Heather had cancer. It had been discovered on a routine doctor visit. It did not look good. I remember hanging up and rejoining my own family of two active teenage girls and a healthy husband, thinking that could have been us. There was a unanimous response: What can we do?

"There were weeks of just waiting for news. We would get an occasional phone call or email. It mostly sounded like a brave front. We were encouraged not to trouble them with calls—they needed their time. We spoke to a friend from church that was an authority on nutrition and a three-time cancer survivor. We got her and Heather connected. More waiting.

"Then our opportunity came. Heather would be in Ann Arbor, at U of M, for several weeks. We sprang into action. This was our turf. I can remember the excitement—multiple weeks in a hospital room with nothing to do. We culled through our video collection for good picks and headed off to a local Blockbuster to buy another stack of recent hits. As I recall, we threw in a few magazines and few nibbles for Larry and headed off to deliver our bounty to her hospital room.

"We were thrilled to get another assignment shortly thereafter. Wow. We had something to do again! This time it was making nutritional smoothies using only fresh, organic ingredients and soymilk. What was soymilk? In Ann Arbor this was no sweat. This time it was my husband that did most of the concocting and then would rush off to the hospital to deliver them while still chilled.

"Looking back, Heather's struggle taught us a lot about patience and persistence. There were times we were about to throw in the towel and figure we were destined to watch this play out from the bleachers. But, we kept nudging and finally got a chance to do something.

"When Heather first wrote her book, we were amazed that our actions were even remembered. Our contributions seemed pretty forgettable. We were wrong. Small things do count. Don't assume there is no role when you ask only once. Be there. Do the stupid stuff. It counts."

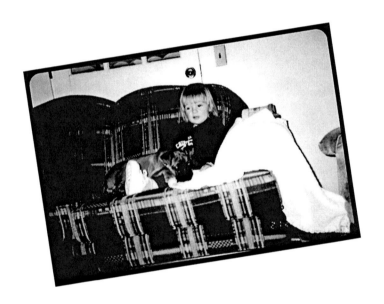

CHAPTER 11

The Setback

Sydney Bs,

I always knew there was a God. I just never thought about how interested He was in me. You know I've been praying a lot lately and I can feel Him closer to me. I feel as though He is helping me find the way and He is providing the people that we need to be OK. Imagine that. God wants to talk with me. I bet that in your life you'll have times of feeling close or far from God but I pray that you'll always know that He loves you, so much that He let His own son die for you. Sometimes it seems hard to hear God, but many times I think we just don't listen. I think He speaks through people and things that happen in our lives if we notice these things. The keyword is "if."

I love you, silly.

Mommy

ARMED WITH NEW confidence, and awed by the God who had brought me through the valley, I was released 19 days after coming to the spa. It was the Monday after Easter, which had been my goal. Larry, Sydney and I went to my mom's house to recover for a few days before heading north.

Almost immediately after I got there I started feeling lousy. I was trying to eat but nothing tasted good. I even tried a glass of milk, which used to be my favorite, but my taste buds were shot from all the chemo. I was guzzling Gatorade to keep from getting dehydrated.

Try as I did, I couldn't keep it together and 24 hours later I passed out on the stairs. I woke up spewing Gatorade all over Larry and myself, something I'm sure neither of us will ever forget. I then tried to convince Larry that I would be just fine and there was no need to call anyone. He promptly called U of M and they told him to bring me in. He was right. I needed to go, but I didn't want to. I had just been freed two days earlier.

It was an interesting day at the Cancer Center. I was pretty dehydrated, which was why I had passed out. Dr. Ayash came in to see me. Again I was begging her, asking not to be re-admitted back to 8A. She cranked up the saline drip and made me a deal. If I could stand up for two minutes without any trouble by the time the Cancer Center closed at 9 p.m., I could go home. If not, welcome back to 8A. I told her that I felt great. I was even eating chicken nuggets and a potato from Wendy's. She smiled and said she couldn't believe I was eating that stuff, meaning most people go for bland, not fried nuggets. I knew it wasn't a great nutritional choice, but I was desperate.

The challenge was on. All afternoon and evening when I thought I could do it, I would call in Chrissy, an aide, and have her time me. Each time I failed, but after a while it was funny—me getting all geared up just to stand for two minutes. It was another example of one of those things you could never think you would laugh at. Then you learn about cancer humor.

I never made the two minute mark, so back I went to lovely 8A. I was greeted by all my nurses who told me that they knew I wasn't ready to leave just a few days earlier.

I spent two horrible nights in the hospital, complete with an annoying roommate. I ate a lot of popsicles, watched *101 Dalmatians* in the middle of the night because I couldn't sleep, and made it my mission to talk to any docs that I could find in the hopes of an early release.

When I did get the ear of two doctors at once, I watched my dream of going home fade in a cruel way. Dr. Uberti was with Dr. Reynolds. Dr. Uberti, being the senior doctor, asked Dr. Reynolds if after reviewing my chart he thought it was OK for me to go home. Dr. Reynolds, being cautious, told me he would like me to stay one more night. Dr. Uberti said that was fine, though he probably would have let me go. Ugh! That was not what I wanted to hear.

After another long night the morning came and I was sitting outside my door waiting for Dr. Ayash when she came round. It was barely 7 a.m. When she saw me waiting in the hall she told me she would come and see me first. She came in and brought a resident with her. While doing my exam she told the resident that I had made remarkable progress, and that she was very pleased. She couldn't have paid me a higher compliment. Dr. Ayash's words have always been few, but meaningful. To top it all off she let me go home.

I left there humbled, once again realizing that I was not in control. I think in some ways I had gotten used to things working in my favor and in my time. This little visit helped me to remember that it may not always be the way I wanted it to be.

Snapshot: Christy, Heather's Best Friend

"I have been asked time and again the best way to help someone who is going through cancer. I think the team approach may be the best advice for caregivers. Being the sole caretaker would be very stressful and taxing. Larry, Colleen and I shared the role—we were a team. Our individual strengths combined to support Heather in different ways. Each of us could also feel good that someone else was there or on their way when we weren't. The situation was never very far from our thoughts, but we could get away and sleep, exercise, relax or eat well, whatever we needed to do to take care of ourselves. A caregiver that gets run down and sick can't be around to help.

"I also get asked how this experience has changed me. I think I got to realize how precious and uncertain life is earlier than I would have. It made me realize we each only get one life. I took that to heart and changed my life in a million ways. I learned to choose *me* sometimes and let go of some of the people in my life who took too much. Life was too short to spend with anyone who left me drained and feeling bad about who I was.

"I went back to school and got my master's degree in exercise science and now I get to work with people every day who are trying to improve their lives through wellness. I understand the importance of the choices I make for myself every day. I know exercising and eating well matters. I live a much more conscious life than I did before.

"I remember the first Thanksgiving after Heather's diagnosis and reflecting over the past year. I realized that that had been the best and worst year of my life. I never thought the best and the worst could be the same year. I had never been so sad or so scared and yet I saw colors, sunshine and the simple joy of being with people I loved more than ever before. I would never wish a cancer diagnosis on anyone, but I know for certain that good things come out of bad things.

"Heather and I have remained closer than ever as friends. We never grow very far apart, even if we don't see each other very often. We have spent many, many hours on the phone. I think we navigate the world together. We run important things and not so important things past each other. She is a compass for me."

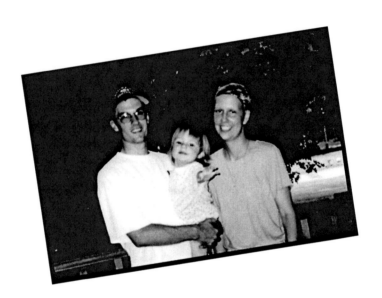

CHAPTER 12

Half Time

Sydney Bs,
My favorite time of year is the spring. I love seeing things growing every day, the leaves coming out on the trees, the tulips and daffodils pushing through the ground for another year. My favorite color is red. I love its vibrancy and its strength. My favorite ice cream flavor is mint chocolate chip, though I shouldn't have it anymore. My favorite car is a Fiat. I almost talked my dad into getting me one. My favorite job was working as a camp counselor, I loved having fun every day, being crazy, singing before every meal. It was the greatest. My favorite wish is that I will know all of your favorites. My favorite girl is you.
Love,
Mommy

AHHH, FREEDOM. I was so glad to be home, but I was far from ready to be on my own. Larry, Sydney and I went back to our home, with my mom coming along to help out for a few days. I was no longer feeling any nausea, but I wasn't ready to resume my normal routine either. I mostly felt like lying around, only getting on my feet to do necessary things. We walked into a clean house, courtesy of the Cooking Girls from church; and our dog had been given a complete checkup and bath, thanks to Karen, Pastor Jim's wife. It took some time to unpack, as I had accumulated so many things while in the hospital. Sydney had also added to her growing collection of toys.

Figuring out our days took a little planning. I wasn't allowed to change messy diapers, due to the possibility of germs causing an infection. Though I could take care of myself, Sydney was a little out of my league energy-wise. We had many offers of babysitting for Syd, but I didn't want her to leave me as I hadn't seen her in some time. Fortunately, Christy came up and stayed. People from church pitched in again and we made it through the first weeks. It left me feeling helpless, sitting on the couch while others vacuumed, made me lunch, and took care of my child. I just kept track of scheduling people. What a humbling time.

Having been on the sidelines for a few weeks was tough, but I decided to view it as a half time of sorts to rest and recharge. I got stronger though and soon it was time to write another letter to my supporters.

> Dear Friends,
> The book of Hebrews warns us to hold on to our confidence and it will be richly rewarded. I haven't thrown my confidence away, but I must say it has faltered in the past weeks. I'm not sure if that is because I spent so much time away from the places that give me strength or because U of M makes cancer their problem and not God's. In any case, now that I am home I'm searching for the

strength and confidence that was once mine. I'm sure that I can find it again.

It is wonderful to be home, to go to baseball games and church, to play outside with Sydney. I thank God that I only had to spend three weeks in the hospital; some on my floor were doing three-month stints. It was also wonderful to be the one with the most mail every day, with prayers being said for me when I was working on just existing, and with food being brought up to me every day that I was actually eating real food. Thank you all for your help in my healing. This truly was a group effort.

In the answered prayers column, my family and I continue to add many things. After contracting pneumonia in the hospital I was given a chest X-ray two days after getting out and it was completely gone. They said I wasn't the same girl. God works swiftly sometimes. I also continue to get letters on a regular basis that start out, "You don't know me but ... " These are the best—feeling as though cancer is making people's faith stronger and encouraging us all to reach out and embrace each other.

For prayer concerns I would ask that you continue to pray for healing, negative test results, and that I will be directed to use this cancer and my life to change other lives. I'm not sure how, but I may have some interesting possibilities. I would also encourage you to pick a few other people who weigh on your heart to talk to God about. Thank you for all the pictures. My scrapbook didn't get very far in the hospital, though, as I was too busy throwing up. If you would still like to send pictures, I have plenty of space to put them in. For those of you who would like a picture of me (bald or with hair), I'd be happy to send you one. Just let me know. I'll continue to keep up my end of the correspondence and would love for you to keep up with me, either through mail or email. Happy spring. Hope you enjoy every sunny day. Have a great day.

Love,

Heather and Larry

With the testing going well, my team and I made plans for round two, the next stem cell transplant. It was approved by my insurance company and would likely be coming up in 3–4 weeks. This one would be outpatient, meaning I would go to the infusion center every day, but could go home (to my parent's house) after each treatment. I was warned that most stem cell patients end up being admitted due to infection or severe mouth pain. My goal was to stay out the whole time. It would be a different set of chemo drugs this time.

There was not a plan for what would happen after the transplant. Surgery was a possibility, as was radiation. Regardless of the future, I knew I needed to be as fit as possible. I resumed walking and eating well. I was taking my supplements and nurturing my soul. As my strength returned, so did my determination. I was ready to begin.

Snapshot: Colleen, Heather's Mother

"I've learned that it's OK to follow your instincts and do things that make sense. We were both completely unimpressed with the nutrition advice we got initially. I found Dr. Block's name in several books and encouraged Heather to call his office. This turned out to be a great resource for all of us. I went to many of her appointments, both because I wanted to know what was happening and because I had read how hard it is for the patient to absorb and remember all that is said. I did a lot of research on the Internet and only told Heather the positive things I found, but could relate some of the other things as they became relevant. I took care of Sydney and drove to the hospital each day during the first stem cell transplant. They stayed at my house for three weeks for the second transplant, which required someone to drive her to Ann Arbor each day while someone else took care of Sydney. I was still working full time through all of this but my boss allowed me to change my schedule around as needed. I did her laundry, bought organic food—whatever I could.

"Heather's cancer made me realize how quickly things can change; how vital your health is; and how many things I do that affect my health. You should appreciate what you have, enjoy every day and don't put off doing things. It's especially important to spend time with people—family and friends. In 2006, my husband was diagnosed with a very rare disease. I retired and we took a trip through New England which he had always wanted to do. A year later, he was using a walker and can't walk at all now. I am so glad we took that trip."

Every day we are killing cancer.

But I will restore you to health and heal your wounds, declares the Lord. Jeremiah 30:17

CHAPTER 13

Round Two

Sydney Bs,

Guess what I have figured out? I am not very patient. It seems like more and more the worst thing for anyone to hear is that they need to wait. I admit I am one of those people. I hope you will be better at it than I am someday. I want you to be the very best of Daddy and me. You will have to work hard, to be persistent (somehow I don't think that will be a problem), to be kind to others, and to believe in yourself. It is so fun to wonder who you will be become. I hope that you will follow your heart and your dreams. Don't believe the naysayers. I know. I can't listen to them either right now. This is a crazy road, but somehow we are making a way. I love you, girl.

Mommy

TRANSPLANT NUMBER TWO started on a Monday this time, May 10. I went to the Cancer Center to have another central line placed, as my other one was removed before I left the "spa." I wasn't nearly as nervous this time and found myself joking with the nurse as she got me ready. Little did I know it was training day, and I was the guinea pig—just one of the many perks of being at a teaching hospital. The doctor performing the placement narrated exactly what he was doing as he taught the second doctor the procedure. It wasn't a big deal at first, but as he was placing the line in my vein it didn't go in as smoothly as before. He suggested to his student that maybe because it had already been done once there was some scar tissue. I was thinking maybe it just wasn't a good day. Either way, hearing each step made it much more painful. This wasn't the start to round two that I had anticipated.

Once punctured and ready to receive fluids, I went to the infusion room where they hooked me up to my chemo. It was Taxol this time, which was put into a fanny pack, since it had to run for 24 hours. I scheduled the time for my return the next day and we left. Christy had accompanied me so we chose to go to out to lunch and shop at Whole Foods, one of our newest favorite stores. There was no reason to waste a good day together. It was the weirdest thing, shopping while getting chemo—one thing so lighthearted, the other so serious. Later, back in our old neighborhood, we spent a nice spring afternoon on the boat. We felt compelled to live and enjoy every day. Though I was bald and hooked up to chemo, I had fun.

The daily treks to Ann Arbor began. The first day for chemo, the second to remove my fanny pack and get fluids. More chemo on day three. This time, at the Cancer Center. On Thursday, I got my stem cells back, without any trouble. This time Larry was there to see it.

My brother Troy, home from Texas, came with me to Ann Arbor one day. He checked out the Cancer Center, and then, God love him, took off to find old friends in the hospital. By the time he returned, I was already done and ready to go home. For what he lacked in companionship that day he more than made up for in managing all my medications. I was taking multiple pills for nausea, heartburn and pain. He made a color-coded chart that we all followed to get them all in on time.

Two days after getting my stem cells back, I was still feeling good, moving around the house and playing with Syd. Her favorite activities involved cooing to her babies and lining them up all in a row. Since it was pretty low key, I could keep up. Even as I began to feel worse, I spent my time lying on the futon in my parent's living room, watching Disney movies with Sydney. There was a Dalmatian movie that was played again and again. To this day just hearing the music brings on feelings of being sick all by itself. But it was better than the hospital.

I was drinking a ton as my throat was really dry and I didn't want to get dehydrated again. My throat kept getting thicker as I began to feel worse. Twenty-four hours later I was throwing up every few minutes on the way to Ann Arbor. I was sure I'd be getting admitted.

God Bless Larry, my mom, and Christy for driving me back and forth to Ann Arbor each day. It was not a fun journey. There were days I was throwing up every few minutes on the way and back. I was always worried that I would have to stay.

One day I also got a blood transfusion. The difference in the way I felt was immediate—more energy and a little spring in my step. It was incredible. I am grateful to the many who donate their blood.

My doctors did a great job of managing my pain and problems. It was because of their amazing care that I made it through the whole thing without spending a night at the hospital. After 13 days I was given the OK to stop the daily trips. I only needed to return at some point to remove my line.

I was the second of 10 stem cell patients to make it through the entire transplant procedure without being admitted. It was an accomplishment that made me proud.

Snapshot: Troy, Heather's Older Brother

"I was in Texas when Heather called and told me that she had a mass in her breast. She told me that she had just had a biopsy and visited the surgeon. As I listened, I was freaking out. I had only been out of medical school for a year and I was thinking of this strictly in terms of what the odds were. I was looking at the research and thinking, *my sister is going to die.* The doctors were not giving her any hope.

"My mom called after Heather talked to the first oncologist. She wanted me to find someone else to be her doctor. I got the next day off of work so I could do something. I began by calling one of my professors at U of M. He gave me Dr. Merajver's name. I was able to talk with her and tell her Heather's story. She promised me that she was going to call Heather immediately and that she would get her in for an appointment in the next week.

"I was initially in shock, but as a physician I wanted to act and get her to the best medical care I could find. I'd like to think I played a part. I also know Heather has played a part in how I practice medicine today.

"As a young physician you don't know what you don't know. I didn't feel uncomfortable providing the basics of what the regimen for Heather's cancer should look like. I could look up literature and find research. However, over my years of practice I have learned that there are a lot of ways to come to an answer that will work for a patient or a family. Experience lends a huge advantage in finding the right choice for each patient.

"I have also learned that a prognosis is just an average. While I can fully recall the lecture in medical school where that was explained, I absolutely understand that now. When you are talking to someone about numbers you have no idea which group they will be in. So the prognostic numbers don't matter. What matters is how people want to live their lives. What do they want to get out of their life? You talk about how to get there. What do they enjoy? What do they fear and want to avoid? It gets a lot easier to make hard decisions regarding medical care and procedures when you know the answers to these questions.

"Heather showed me that it is very important to know what matters to my patients. If I know what they are trying to get out of their life we can work to get there. There are lots of choices. If I knew then what I know now, I would have had more hope for Heather when we first talked.

"There are two experiences that I recount with patients on a regular basis. One is working on a farm where I learned that only when you are done with your chores can you have fun. That helps me relate to the people I treat in rural Michigan. The other experience that helps me is Heather's. I understand better now that every person is different, and so is every situation. God wants us to trust Him and trust that He is going to participate in our lives.

"Heather's diagnosis has helped me be a far better doctor."

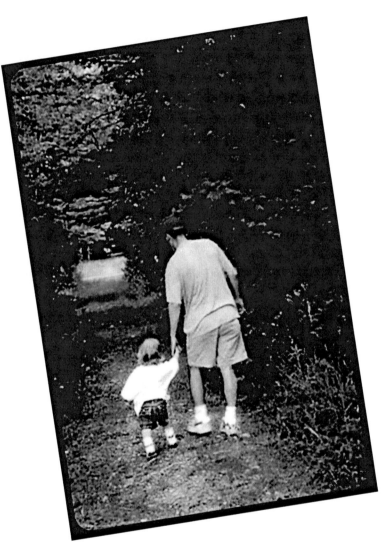

CHAPTER 14

The New Me

Sydney Bs,

Here is my advice on dating:

1. You can't fool Daddy and me; don't even try.

2. Be too busy sometimes; a little chase is good for everyone.

3. Be yourself; after all, that is who you will always be.

4. Don't settle for OK; find the one who makes your heart sing.

5. When you are happy with who you are it shows, and people will be attracted to you.

6. Dream big.

7. Know that no one, not even Prince Charming, will be good enough in your daddy's eyes. What an amazing thought to think that someday you'll be all grown up.

I love you,

Mommy

AFTER THE TRANSPLANT, I took time to regain my strength and enjoy my family. This brought us through the month of June. It had been six months. During that time, we made another trip to The Block Center in Evanston to visit with doctors and the dietitian. David, the dietitian, was a constant source of encouragement and motivation for me. He reinforced what I was doing nutritionally and always had suggestions to help me overcome the side effects of treatment.

I scheduled surgery for a double mastectomy right after the July Fourth weekend. The decision to have a double mastectomy was left up to me, but I did not need to consider it for long. The answer was clear to me. I was anxious to stay on track and finish treatment as soon as possible. I knew my husband's football season was coming quickly.

We spent a sunny Fourth of July weekend with friends out on their boat. It was great to relax and hang out, with a minimal amount of cancer talk. Matt and Joy put me at ease and we left feeling refreshed.

I came to realize that it isn't an easy task to act natural around someone facing a serious illness like mine. People tend to censor themselves in one of two ways: either they act it was as if laughing is no longer allowed, or they pretend that life is just a bowl of cherries. Matt and Joy hit the balance perfectly.

I went back to Ann Arbor for the mastectomy with a good attitude.

My surgery was scheduled for the morning of July 5. After saying goodbye to Sydney and leaving her with Larry's parents, we set off for U of M once again. Today we were going to a part of the hospital that was new to me. After parking and walking into the main hospital entrance, we found a large room for the people waiting to have surgery. I checked in and was told to have a seat. It was fairly full in the room but we found a spot to wait for my turn. I looked about and found myself wondering what all these people were here for. I had never thought of surgery as a planned event, just something you might be rushed in for unexpectedly. By the look of this place however, it seemed as though a lot of people planned ahead.

Time passed and we waited. My scheduled time came and went, and after a while my surgeon, Dr. Pass, came and found us in the waiting room. She was running behind, but not worried. She assured me I would be in that afternoon. I was glad for a chance to talk with her. Dr. Pass was the kind of doctor who spoke to you as if she was your friend, not as the director of the Breast Care Clinic at a major university hospital. I wanted to be sure she knew about my choice to have a double mastectomy. She understood my fears and concerns. I told her I felt it was the right choice for me and that Larry fully supported it.

I had one more thing that had been weighing on my mind. I told her that if she found cancer she was not to panic. I wanted no negative energy in the operating room. She surprised me by nodding enthusiastically. I knew she understood.

With that said I felt at ease. We spent the afternoon playing cards—Larry and my parents—as if we were just hanging out at home. I was finally called in at 4 p.m. to get ready for surgery.

When I was first diagnosed with the cancer my initial reaction was that I wanted it out—*now*. I was surprised to find surgery would come later. But as I went through the chemo and could actually see the changes in my breast as the tumor shrank, it was incredibly reassuring. If I had had surgery first, I wouldn't have seen the progress I had already made to this point. I wasn't emotionally wrought over losing a part of my body. In fact, I saw it in a positive light, such as no more bras. I guess more than anything I felt that losing my breasts was a small price to pay for life.

My surgery went smoothly and though I didn't get into the operating room until 5:45 p.m., I was done by 8:30. They had estimated four to six hours, but hadn't needed that much time. Tissue and lymph nodes were sent to be biopsied to determine if there were any cancer cells.

I spent the night and called Christy early the next morning asking for a shake. She was happy to oblige my request and to hear that I felt like eating. When she came up to my room I asked her if she wanted to see my chest. I was amazed at the way it looked, because it seemed almost normal to me. Just a flat chest. Nothing more, nothing less. I was amazed and thankful once again that I had found such an amazing surgeon who had taken great care of me. The grossest part of the procedure were the ugly drains for the excess fluid. I had all of my lymph nodes removed on the left side, so I needed two drains on that side. The right side only had one. The drains repulsed me, even after everything I had been through. I couldn't wait for them to come out.

Feeling good, though sore, I was released that afternoon, less than 24 hours after going into the OR. I went back to my parents for a few days to recover. Two days later, I had two of the drains taken out and six days after surgery, the final one was removed. I was pleased with my progress. We headed back to our home.

The hardest part about having the surgery was Sydney. I would have given anything for her to understand why I couldn't pick her up. A 10-pound weight limit and a 20-pound daughter just don't mesh. It broke my heart as we taught her to climb up the step stool and into her crib so that I could then put the rail up and she could sleep as always. I would cajole and beg her to walk with me instead of being carried. It felt as though the cancer was now affecting her and that angered me. Hurting me was one thing, but leave my daughter alone. As much as I wanted to be near Sydney or she wanted to climb on me and snuggle close, it was too painful. We found if we put a pillow between us I could read to her and it pacified us both.

Within a week or so I was back to walking and as active as always, with the exception of the month-long weight limitation. Dr. Merajver and I met again and she felt I should have radiation. This would be my last phase of treatment. The new me was ready.

Snapshot: Kim, Larry's Sister

"Want to feel totally helpless? Hear by phone that, two states away, your baby brother's young wife—the mother of your brand new niece—has cancer. The bad kind. The really, really bad kind. Want to make it worse? Go to Google and start typing in terms like 'stage IV.'

"It's hard to remember what I felt exactly, except for shock, upon learning of my sister-in-law Heather's diagnosis and nasty prognosis. You know how you never know what to say to someone facing something like this? It's equally hard, or perhaps more so, to know what you can *do*, particularly when geography keeps you from being close enough to make casseroles, drive to appointments or even help with house cleaning or child care. What I knew I couldn't do is let materialize the awful images that popped into my head of my brother raising this adorable baby who'd just taken her first steps, alone—without his beloved.

"At the time, my good friend Debbie was making table fountains. In each, she'd place at least one rock shaped like a heart, a treasure she'd scour beaches for throughout the year. Debbie is someone who, like a fountain, bubbles over with joy, even on her worst days. She is also a counselor and spiritual director and seemingly more tapped into God and healing powers than anyone I know. Her fountains, then, represented more than the relaxation and stress reduction I wanted to provide with a gift. They were about healing and hope. So that's what I sent off via a UPS truck—a tiny trickle of hope that would join the prayers and kindnesses of many others to become a full-blown healing stream."

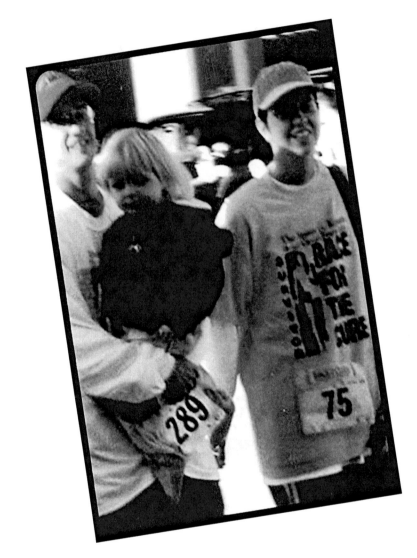

CHAPTER 15

Nearing the Finish Line

Sydney Bs,

I have learned that we should never stop learning in our lives. I have been learning so much lately, about my walk with God, about food, about balance. I have no idea where that is going to take us, so for now I am just trying to move forward. I never expected the changes that we have had this year, but that's OK. We can handle whatever comes our way. Some days I am afraid of the future, other days I can't wait. I guess that is the key—to live in the moment and yet be mindful of the future. Or to be grateful for what we have and yet always strive for the very best that life has to offer. Or maybe I still have a lot left to learn. Either way, I love you.

Mommy

THE PREPARATION FOR radiation began. I had the range of motion needed in my left arm, meaning I could raise and keep my arm above my head. That was necessary in order to do radiation. Before starting though, I had to make a decision about my job. My medical leave had only been granted through June. I had to look at whether or not I could go back to work in the fall and maintain the regime that I felt was crucial to staying healthy. I chose, with my husband's support, to resign. Radiation would have extended into the school year by about a month and I knew I wasn't ready to try to juggle it all.

Larry, my mom and I began to map out what my radiation would look like. Dr. Lori Pierce was to oversee my radiation in Ann Arbor. Aside from a long list of national awards, she was just plain nice. After meeting with her and discussing options, we all agreed that it would be better for me to receive the radiation in Lansing. This would save me two hours of driving each day. U of M had a partnership there, so Dr. Pierce could oversee the treatments.

I was pushing to get things moving quickly as July was fading fast and August in our house means two things: football and an absentee husband. This isn't a derogatory statement, it is simply the truth. We don't see a lot of Larry during football. I have never minded his annual absence, but I knew this year it might be a challenge with all I was facing.

I began in Lansing by meeting my new doctor, another woman, and having more tests done. The plan was to do radiation to the left chest region, as reoccurrence tends to happen at the original breast cancer site. My tissue samples from the surgery had come back clean, with no sign of cancer cells, so the radiation was just another punch to keep the cancer from returning.

The treatment was set for 30 sessions. I would be going to Lansing five days a week for six weeks. After the testing and a discussion with my doctor, I met with three radiation techs. I assumed this would be a simple process.

They began with a mold of my body so that I could be positioned in the exact same spot each day. The process turned out to be almost more than I could handle emotionally. They had me lie on my back on a table with my shirt off. Without warning, they whipped out their sharpies and began to draw across my now-breastless chest. They joked that they were just doing a little art. What they called artwork, along with their insensitive comments, were capped off by orders not to shower so that they could see their "masterpiece" the next day. It was horrible.

Still shirtless, I was told I would be getting permanent tattoos across my chest as landmarks for the radiation. I wanted to know why, how big they would be and how many. I managed to slow them down and make them talk to me. After some serious negotiations, we agreed to two small dots—one on my upper chest and one below my armpit. Neither would be bigger than the tip of a sharpened pencil.

That day I made a vow. If I ever worked in healthcare, I would know my patients as individuals, beyond their diagnosis. I was tired of being called a "CT scan" or whatever test I was having. I was tired of having things minimized and made light of. I was tired of being dehumanized in the eyes of those doing the testing. Each patient is part of a family who loves them. I would not make light of their situation for my benefit. I would remember what it feels like to be the patient, and honor the feelings of anxiety and fear.

My radiation treatments began on the same day Larry started football practice. Bring on the busy season. It was a massive coordination nightmare. I had arranged for someone to watch Sydney every morning. Then the radiology scheduler told me that I would have to come in the afternoon, as mornings were filled. I said no, it had to be mornings. By this time I was putting my foot down. I was not in the mood to negotiate. I just wanted it done. It got done.

Radiation has a tendency to make people tired so I scheduled to have drivers as many days as possible. In order to get volunteer drivers we made a calendar that said "Driving Miss

Heather" at the top. We passed it through the pews at church. Those sitting the closest to us all got a chance to take an exciting trip to Lansing; estimated time of trip—four hours. Fortunately, by the end of the service, most time slots were filled. I only had a few to figure out on my own.

So it began. I would get up, take Sydney to daycare and come back to meet my driver to go to Lansing. Once there, I would wait in the patient waiting room, which always had a jigsaw puzzle on the table to work. A great idea, I must say, as it helped pass the time, and if they were running behind I never really cared.

The radiation itself took about two minutes. I would lie on the table, positioned in my mold and the techs would leave the room. I would lie still while the machine would rotate to the three different angles. Buzz, buzz, buzz, see you tomorrow.

I ran into a stumbling block the end of my first week of radiation. I was having some itching in my hairline—what little there was of it. It felt like a tiny pimple that wouldn't pop. I saw the doctor after my treatment on Friday. He told me it was shingles. I had no idea what that was. The doc called U of M and they wanted me to be sent to Ann Arbor for further evaluation. Shingles is a form of the chicken pox virus, and very common after a transplant due to a weakened immune system. The virus was located in the left upper quadrant of my head, and possibly in my eye, where it could cause blindness. Off I went to be evaluated at U of M.

By the time I got there it was Friday afternoon. I missed the doctor who put in PICC lines, so that eliminated the ability to have the drugs at home with a visiting nurse. I ended up being admitted for the weekend so I could be on IV antibiotics. I was released on Monday, ready to start back with the radiation.

The folks in Lansing said that because I was contagious the morning appointments I had fought so hard for would not be possible. I could expose someone else to shingles. I was made to come in the late afternoon. At U of M I had been told that once I was on medication I was no longer contagious, but Lansing didn't buy that. My daycare schedule was in chaos and I was feeling the same.

A week or so later I was able to return to my morning spot. As I chatted with a gentleman I had met earlier, I told him about the shingles. He shared that he had been dealing with shingles since before my outbreak. No one made him change his time. I wondered if he exposed me to begin with. I was questioning my choice to radiate in Lansing.

Aside from the shingles, I was doing well. Every week I would meet with the radiation doctor who had warned me that I would have second to third degrees burns on the radiation sites. So I called the Block Center, the Evanston docs and nutrition experts and they suggested changes to my diet and special supplements to take. As a result of this, my skin barely turned pink throughout the radiation.

I was not as compatible with the radiation staff as I had been with all of my other docs. We were on different pages. After one appointment I was offered candy from a dish on the counter. I said, "No thanks, sugar feeds cancer." I saw heads shake and I knew I was too intense for them.

I may have been approaching the finish line but this last stretch was tough. A few weeks into radiation I began having trouble with lightheadedness. Glenna, a good soul and a Texas princess living in The North, came to pick me up for one of my trips to Lansing. She opened the front door and found me lying on the floor. I hadn't passed out, but I couldn't sit up without blacking out. Glenna, in "go-big-or-go-home" Texas-fashion was ready to call in the National Guard or at least an ambulance. I asked for a glass of orange juice and told her I'd be ready in a minute. Once I had the juice, I was upright and ready to go. I'm not sure Glenna was the same. Learning from this experience, I began to have Larry put a glass of OJ on the nightstand for me to drink before I tried to move in the morning. It worked.

As we approached the end of my radiation, Larry and I saw a TV promotion for the Race for the Cure. We decided to walk it.

I set a goal to run it the following year. I sent out a letter asking for pledges and $1,100 came in over the next week.

I was still in radiation when we went to the race early in September. It was the first time I was honored as a survivor. I had mixed feelings of pride and humility, as well as joy and sadness. The event was awesome. The walk itself was interesting, with many people cheering us on. Poor Larry ended up carrying Sydney almost the whole way as she refused to sit in her stroller, but we finished with smiles and a good feeling in our hearts. I started this race in treatment and finished it as a survivor.

I finished radiation on a Tuesday, jumping for joy that I was done. Besides the shingles, which had impacted the nerves in my forehead, I was no worse than when I had started. I realize now I was never as invested in the radiation as I was in my earlier treatments. I still wonder if it was really necessary at all. As a cancer patient, I was willing to do anything I was offered, though. If I walked that path again, I am not sure I would have done the radiation. I have learned how important it is to follow your instincts.

Snapshot: Grandpa Larry, Larry's Father

"There is no preparing for bad news like cancer in your family. Carole and I went to Larry and Heather's house to watch Sydney for what was supposed to be a mundane doctor visit in Grand Rapids. It is all a blur now. When they came home and shared the news, I know I went into shock. I felt all emotion drain from me. I was in disbelief. How could this happen?

"We were numb all the way home. Carole was stronger than I was but we were both struggling. There had to be a mistake. This couldn't be happening. Something must be wrong.

"Then the treatments started. All we could do was try to help. We spent most of our time and effort just trying to update friends and family. We felt pretty helpless. We wrote the updates as much for us as we did for others. It was our way to highlight the milestones, the progress and any good news we could pass along. We didn't want to pass along bad news because we didn't want to hear it.

"Carole handled the one-on-one questions from others. I could sit in front of a keyboard and beat out a news update. I couldn't do the questions.

"Larry and I never talked about how we were feeling. We stayed on safe ground with updates. He was strong and I didn't want to touch that. He needed to stay strong for Heather, for Sydney and for the rest of us.

"We all held our breath. We have talked very little about it until now, almost out of fear. This was a very scary time.

"I look back now on all that Heather has done to help other people. So many people feel hopeless when they get a cancer diagnosis. Her work has given them hope—a place to start; a path to try to take control.

"One other wonderful outcome of all this was Ty's adoption. We had a celebration when he came home at last. It was a wonderful outcome from this terrible time."

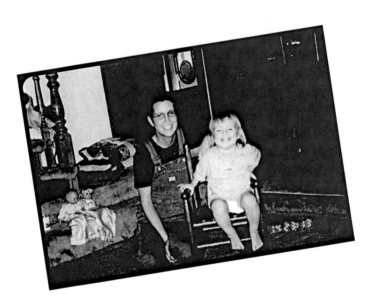

CHAPTER 16

What Now?!

Sydney Bs,

What do you do when you are scared? I always talk to Daddy. He's so good at putting things in perspective. Being scared is OK sometimes. It motivates us to do things that we might not do if everything were OK. It teaches us that we all need each other. I've been scared a lot lately. I'm wondering if the cancer is really gone; if I can move forward in my life. I don't know if I'll be OK without doing some kind of treatment. I don't know who I am anymore. Oh that's right, Sydney's mom. I'll start with that. Thank God for you.

Love,

Mommy

TEN MONTHS AFTER my diagnosis of breast cancer, I completed my last treatment. I marked the end with a letter to the masses.

> To My Faithful Friends,
> Ahhh, it's over, I'm done, finished, complete. I think I have done every treatment they could think of for killing breast cancer.
> It's beautiful outside. The fall colors are brilliant. Our house faces an asparagus field that is a bright yellow with a tree line behind showing all sorts of reds, yellows and greens. With the changing of the trees, my focus will also change. I'm going to learn how to meditate. Survivors generally rank this as the most important change in their lives after cancer. I'm going to make my body strong, physically. I set up a program with a trainer today at a wellness center near my home. I'm going to eat well every day. I will be starting on a detox program to rid my body of residual chemicals and toxins which make functioning more difficult. I will spend quiet time every day with God and I will journal my thoughts. Aside from that, I will try to be a good mom to my great daughter, a good football wife to my husband, and a dedicated youth leader to an exceptional youth group. I feel as though there is a lot on my plate, but it is all positive. Who could ask for more?
> Many of you haven't heard from me in some time. I don't have to be back in Ann Arbor until the end of November, praise God!! At that time, a complete check will be done, and hopefully a report of no cancer once again. These checks will occur at least twice a year.

So, now it's God and me and we're gonna hold off this monster that we call cancer. I'm going to see my baby go to kindergarten; I want the opportunity to adopt another child someday. We have hearts full of love; we're hoping that God shows us the children that need it the most. The Psalms say that when you're afraid, trust in God. That is what this is about now—trusting and having confidence that it can be done.

I thank you all for your tremendous support; I know it will continue through your prayers. We've learned a lot about life and how precious it is. I hope that you have, too. I'm not sure I'm qualified to give advice but I'd challenge each of you to make your own life better every day, in little ways. The little things sure make a difference. I'll be sending a Christmas card—you won't believe all the hair on my head. I hope to hear from you, too.

God be with you,

Heather

Cancer had taken my world and turned it upside down. What was I supposed to do now? It had shown me the mountains and the valleys and now I was supposed to start living a normal life again. I knew I needed to keep the good things and build from there. I wanted to be devoted to wellness, to family and to awareness of the world around me. I didn't realize how many challenges there would be.

As happy as I was to be done, I didn't realize how much I relied on treatments to help me feel as though I was killing cancer. I had used them as a backup plan for days that I didn't eat well; or I would think about it when I was feeling pain somewhere. Now that the crutch was gone, I found it to be quite scary. Some days I was on top of the world, feeling sure that the miracle was complete and I was healed of cancer. Other days

I felt sure that the pain in my back was certainly cancer and I dove into my healing notebook for support as I prayed.

I was also having trouble figuring out how to define *me*. When anyone asked what I was doing now that my treatment was over, I wasn't sure what to say. I didn't think that "trying to stay healthy" was an acceptable answer, although that was the truth. I was not accustomed to saying that I was a stay-at-home mom either. Honestly, Sydney was a piece of cake to take care of. Many people expected that I would be returning to my life as it was before the cancer. I wasn't able to do that. Too much had happened; too many things had changed. I felt that the pre-cancer normal that I had come from did nothing to keep my body strong physically or otherwise. I didn't want to return to that.

Step by step I moved forward, establishing new routines. I was going to the wellness center, continuing to work on eating well, and getting more involved in church. Some days, Sydney and I would go up to the high school to visit Larry. It was a process, but it was really good for me.

Another hurdle that I had to address was that of making future plans. Before the cancer, I had laid out plans for my entire life. However, with the diagnosis, those plans were gone. To attempt to make plans again felt like tempting fate. I finally took the leap and bought plane tickets for Florida for Christmas vacation. It scared me knowing I would have to clear a complete checkup between the purchase and the actual flight. I knew that my life could be turned upside down with each visit to the doctor.

One constant in my new life was Christy. We continued to communicate daily. Throughout the time that I was fighting cancer, Christy was dealing with a marriage that was falling apart. While my treatment was complete, the horrible process of ending the marriage was just beginning for her. Christy was choosing to stand up for herself and we knew she was doing the right thing, but that didn't make it any easier. My struggle was with cancer, hers was with claiming a future for herself.

The bright spot in the struggle was that Christy was spending time at her grandmother's house, which was less than an hour away. We would get together regularly. With Christy, I could be the emerging me and we could bounce between heavy cancer talk and having fun. It was good for both of us as we moved forward.

Christy and I had both learned lessons. We were no longer the same people as when we started out. We didn't want to be, but it often made us feel as though we were living in a foreign land. Dealing with others was strange. The constant complaints about little things that I would hear from people drove me crazy. I found myself wanting to tell everyone they should be focusing on all the good things that a day could bring.

My outlook on life had changed. Thankfully, Larry and I continued to grow closer through it all. I'm not sure I could ever adequately thank him for accepting the changes in me with the grace and ease that he did.

I remember my dad telling me years ago that he liked Larry because he was the first man I had dated that I didn't have to take care of. He was right. I didn't have to take care of him, he could do it himself. If he didn't want what I had made for dinner, he would make something for himself, never saying a word. He was happy to help me set goals and reach them, throwing in laughter along the way. I don't know if I could have supported him through my illness and devoted the same amount of commitment to healing. Instead we were able to be there for each other and draw from our strengths—"Team Jose."

Snapshot: Keri, the Kid Who Found Me

"The hardest thing for me to do (besides math equations or riding a unicycle) is to describe Heather and how I know her. She kind of shifts into the category I need (or she needs) at the time. Sometimes a church friend, a girlfriend, a teacher, an emergency contact or even a parent. Always though, she is my coach. It has been nearly a decade since I have addressed her as anything else. To me, a nickname has never fit someone more perfectly; and since I did my duty and called her by her birth name once in this statement, I will now revert back to calling her 'Coach.'

"I first got to know Coach after she started coming to our high school cross-country practices. My guess is that her cancer had something to do with it, because I doubt a cross-country workout is something a typical adult would attend unless they had an important reason to. She was there running with us all the time, always with a bandana on her head, sometimes with cute little Sydney in tow, never with a complaint. I got used to her presence there, and at church.

"Volleyball, though, was where Heather became Coach to me. She wasn't always an easy coach to have. You do *not* want to lose a game when your coach is a cancer survivor—giving up isn't really their thing. We built our relationship first on hard work, then respect. But behind all that, there was something softer, more intense. Prayers before games. Dinners at her house. Cookie-decorating with her kids. Knowing that when things were about to explode at my home, it would be OK to go on a four-mile walk with Coach and tell her everything. Once that trust was opened up, she transformed into a new kind of coach. My family coach, giving me nothing but love and unflinching support. Showing me what family really means.

"She helped me get through my last year of high school and first year of college, during a time when everything seemed hopeless. With her help, I really thought I had conquered the world; beat my own 'cancer' that took the shape of problems at home instead of cells in my body. And then I was in an auto accident that left me with a little head injury and a lot of depression. This was when Heather stepped her coaching up a notch.

"Those first weeks after my accident, I recovered at Coach's house. I didn't only eat, sleep and take my medicine *because* of her—I did it *for* her. That blend of love and respect I had for Coach made me want to fight like her. Sometimes things were better, and sometimes they were bleak. I do not know how

many times I had been in the hospital where I would be cling-
ing to a little scrap of paper or a nurse's words that said, 'Your
coach called.' I might have been angry and refused visitors or
phone calls, but Coach was always there. Knowing that was
always enough for me.

"She is still always there. It is still always enough for me. Now
that the dust has settled, I am becoming the strong, happy adult
Coach promised I would someday be. Our relationship is a little different. As fellow conquerors, we get to enjoy one another's
successes and joys. We get to celebrate her 40th birthday and
my wedding this year. Instead of swapping tears and late-night
panic calls or emails, I plan on swapping her knitting lessons
for quilting tips.

"I absolutely believe I wouldn't have survived if Coach hadn't.
Not only that, but I wouldn't have gotten through my strug-
gles if she hadn't gone through hers. I wouldn't have met her
if she hadn't been fighting her fight on the cross-country trail
and in church. I wouldn't have accepted her love or her help
if she hadn't lived through something that made her so loving
and helpful. I got to piggyback off her survival, and that is not
something I take lightly. She's my coach for life."

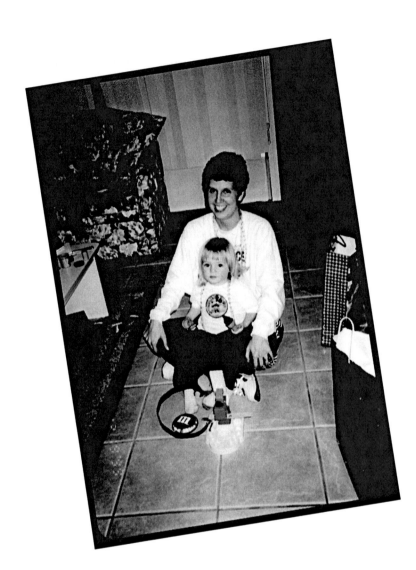

CHAPTER 17

Blessings

Sydney Bs,
"You are my sunshine, my only sunshine, you make me happy when skies are gray ... " What a beautiful girl you are. We have survived the battle. Now if we can just keep on surviving. You are growing so fast, becoming a little girl, cooing to your babies, cooking with the girls. One day you'll be all grown up. I will always love you. I will always be proud of you. I will always be amazed that God blessed me with you. Reach for the stars Sydney Bs. Follow God and make your mark on this old world.
Hugs,
Mommy

EVERY CANCER PATIENT can vividly recall his or her first post-treatment checkup. Mine came in November, just before Thanksgiving. I had no idea how stressful the week would be between doing the test and getting the results. I needed a lot of reassurance as I wavered back and forth on whether or not the cancer was really gone. The tests looked fine. That means that there were no tumors according to a CT scan of my chest, abdomen and pelvis. A few weeks later the bone scan came back stable as well.

This is the point at which I learned about living from appointment to appointment. With good results I was free to move forward with my dreams. As the next appointment approached, the cycle would start again. Stress, fear, relief. Though this has gotten better, it still continues today. I am acutely aware that the results of these appointments can send my life back to the world of cancer.

With the first checkup behind me, the holiday preparations were so much fun with a toddler in the house. Sydney, age 2, had such a sense of awe over every little Christmas tradition. I loved seeing it from her eyes. We had the chance to see her in her first Christmas program at church. Dressed as an angel, she sang every song from her heart. Awesome.

As we boarded the plane to Florida, we looked forward to resuming our yearly tradition at Christmas. This year, though, we cherished our sunshine in December even more. The time spent at our condo with family and friends all together helped us to recall great memories and look forward to building more.

As the rest of the world fretted over the new millennium, I rejoiced that I was here to see it. It seemed fitting to leave the treatment behind in a different century. I was ready to focus on the truths and understandings that life with stage IV cancer had brought me.

It seems to me that there is a cancer in everyone's life, though it does not always come with, "you have six months to live" attached. The crazy thing is that out of those cancers can come the sweetest most meaningful moments in our lives.

The kind words of a stranger, the embrace of your spouse, the laughter of a child are all chances to live in the good moments. On our wedding day, the minister's final prayer for us was that God would give us enough challenges to keep us walking with Him. Although there were many times when I thought back on that with mixed feelings, I've learned to thank God for the challenges.

It will always be challenging for me to deal with the reality that I am here in spite of dismal odds. My cancer was advanced to the point of being terminal. To have the opportunity to continue to parent my child and be a wife is a miracle—plain and simple. I do not know why. I hesitate to claim that God chose me. Sometimes I wonder if it were not for the many people praying for me, if I would even be here. I do strongly feel that my conviction to move quickly and make changes hedged the bets in my favor.

The thought of having cancer will always remain. The reminders are everywhere. I've found that it is necessary to continue to be vigilant about the way that I take care of my body. Every day I am killing cancer. It is not just a sometimes thing. Although I hold myself responsible on a daily basis, were it not for a team of people helping me I don't know where I would be today. Though I can and do make a difference each day, my greatest asset is the people who have helped me succeed.

This is not what I had envisioned for my life, but in many ways, it is better. My experience with cancer has made me dig within myself to look for what God may have planned for me rather than what I had planned for myself. I know that I am living on God's time, but when thinking about that, I realize that we all are.

I wasn't very far into my journey before people were telling me that I should write a book. They had read the letters, which began simply to relay information, with a desire for more. Little did they know that I had been writing letters on my own to Sydney in case things didn't turn out the way that I had hoped.

It became clear to me that I needed to put it all together with the goal that I could make a difference for someone else.

Every day we are killing cancer. You can too!

Snapshot: Bev, Editor of *Breast Cancer Wellness* **Magazine**

"It might be an odd thing to say, but I truly believe I was led to meet Heather. I wanted to add a new contributing writer for the *Breast Cancer Wellness* magazine; not someone who had clinical training in breast cancer, but someone who had personally experienced this life-threatening disease and who had life-saving messages for the readers of the magazine.

"I used the Internet to seek an empowered young woman. I found myself in a website that had mind-boggling, long lists of young women facing breast cancer. Intuitively, I felt directly connected to the name of Heather Jose, yet I didn't know a thing about her, what she looked like or what her story was. One of the most valuable lessons I have learned through this experience of breast cancer is that one of our greatest gifts is intuition. Lo and behold, intuition is what brought me the perfect messenger and role model for healing.

"Not only did Heather understand what the *Breast Cancer Wellness* magazine was about, but here she was, a young mother who had been given a six-month death sentence in 1998 by a professional medical doctor.

"Heather uses her life every day to empower herself and to lead others to commit themselves to do something daily for their wellness experiences. Her message is consistent: Do something every day to strengthen your well-being and have a team who believes in wellness and thriving and who helps to hold you accountable and stay focused on the healing track.

"This may sound too simple to be effective, but Heather has defied her odds by doing simple life-strengthening things every day. She doesn't hang around pity partiers, naysayers or doctors who do not believe in her healing efforts.

"When others unconsciously try to sidetrack Heather from her objectives, she automatically returns to her healing team who helps keep 'thriving' in the forefront. It is the only goal.

"We can all learn from Heather's life-saving messages."

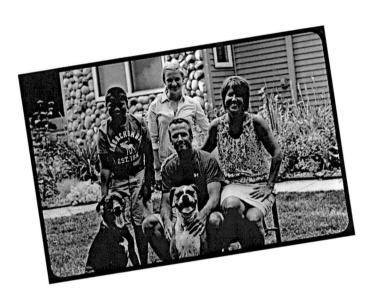

Afterword

I NOW HAVE had many reports that my cancer is stable. I am often asked if I am in remission, but that is not the way it works with bone mets. The goal would be no progression. Anytime I hear that, I am happy. I would like to be able to treat my cancer as if it is a chronic condition rather than a disease. That means continued vigilance and care for my body in order to maintain the high quality of life that I have. There have been a few bumps in the road. We found a spot on my orbit (bone around my eye) and were concerned about one on my spine. Each time, we have been able to switch a med or two and continue. I have not had to do any chemo since my initial treatment, however I continue on a regimen of drugs to this day. I feel like the longer I live, the more I get to enjoy time with my family and the more time I give researchers to come up with something amazing. It is a give and take. I will do all that I can, but I may need some help from conventional medicine from time to time.

There have been other milestones since cancer became the norm in our house. I reached my 30th birthday, a benchmark for me. I celebrated by walking the Avon Breast Cancer 3-Day in Chicago with Christy and my college roommate, Katie. While on the last mile of our walk, I received a phone call that changed our lives. Our son, Ty, born in India and placed in our family with God's faithful help, was ready to come home. He is a gift, and if it took cancer to find him it was all worth it. The adoption process is another book in itself, but let me just thank Sharin for being so persistent.

I reached my very first goal of watching my daughter go to kindergarten, bawling as she rode away on the bus to begin her first day in Chris Cotton's class. Ty was with me as we watched her go and I have to say it really threw me for a loop. However, in time, I a set a new goal and found a routine to carry on.

I spoke about the double mastectomy earlier in my book. At the time, I could have cared less about having reconstructive surgery. I didn't want to slow down the healing process by doing an additional procedure. A few years after my mastectomy, I changed my mind and pursued the reconstruction. I was tired of clothes not fitting right. The process was a difficult one, and I am really glad that I waited to do it. I am happy with the results, though, and would tell anyone that it was worth the pain.

Almost immediately after I finished my treatment, I began to receive invitations to speak at cancer celebrations and the like. Over time, that has grown into a business and a few years ago I officially started "Go Beyond Treatment." I chose the name because I want people in the medical community (patients and their caregivers too) to realize that a treatment is only one piece of the puzzle as we seek to heal. There are other things beyond treatment that impact the healing process. I want to empower patients to feel that they can make a difference in their own bodies. There is nothing I love more than killing cancer and teaching others to do the same. My goal is to help healthcare providers realize that a great patient experience makes an empowered patient. I also want to encourage patients to be the captain of their wellness team in and out of the healthcare setting.

As for my daily life, it is in some ways similar and other ways vastly different than it was when I wrote this book. There isn't a day that goes by that doesn't involve cancer in some way. I'm OK with that, especially if it is because I feel I am making a difference. It certainly isn't my singular focus, though. Larry is still a teacher and football coach as well as being a great dad and husband. We have had some great times as a family, and look forward to many more. Christy and I continue our friendship, though most of it is through phone calls. It doesn't matter to either of us how we keep in touch as long as we do. I will always be on a quest to eat well and exercise. Though I am not always as vigilant as I once was, it continues to be a priority for me. Life, at this point is about balancing the needs of my family, my health and my work. I strive to stay in the moment and enjoy what comes. My kids are growing like crazy. Rather than playing with toys, we are often discussing colleges and running to sporting events.

Most recently, as we were putting the finishing touches on this revision, I turned 40. I celebrated with a party at my house with many of the same people that were mentioned in this book. There was no over-the-hill theme for me. We all know that the very fact that we are here is a cause for celebration. I will never know why I am still here when others pass away from cancer. Those are not easy issues for people like me. I do know though that I will do my best to make the most of each day, knowing that it is a gift.

Where Are They Now?

JOSH, HEATHER'S YOUNGER brother, is a CPO (certified prosthetist/orthotist) in Indiana. He also speaks regularly to audiences about orthotics. He and his wife, Brooke, have three children.

Larry, Heather's husband, is a teacher and the head football coach at Chippewa Hills. He continues to be her coach as well.

Marnie, Heather's PT co-worker, is a physical therapist. She continues to affect the lives of individuals through her unwavering support in difficult times.

Dr. Merajver, Heather's U of M doctor, is now the head of Global Health at the University of Michigan. She continues to lead Heather's care medically.

Colleen, Heather's mother, splits her time between Northern and Southern Michigan in order to spend time with and be the caregiver for her husband and mother. In her free time she likes to spend time with her six grandchildren.

Christy, Heather's best friend, is now an exercise physiologist. Her passion is helping others achieve wellness. She and her husband, Jeff, just celebrated five years of marriage.

Mike, a minister in the United Methodist Church, and **Beth,** Heather's neighbors and friends, are pastoring in Central Michigan. They have also become grandparents, a job that Beth is meant for!

David Grotto, Heather's dietitian, is the author of several books including *101 Foods That Could Save Your Life.* He is a nationally known dietitian.

Aunt Kathy MacDonald, Larry's aunt, helped in editing and assembling the final manuscript for *Every Day We Are Killing Cancer,* especially in gathering the many voices of family and friends who share their perspectives in the book. Kathy is the head of the Macdonald Group, a consulting firm based in a historic neighborhood within downtown Ann Arbor, Michigan. Since 1991, her specialty has been helping a wide range of corporate clients meet critical competitive challenges. Kathy might be called a corporate caregiver. She travels widely to help clients who are facing tough changes in the culture, in global markets and in relationships among staff.

Troy, Heather's older brother, is a partner of Hospitalists of Northern Michigan. He also speaks to hospitalists on a regular basis. Troy and his wife, Sibel, have one daughter.

Kim, Larry's sister, is living with her husband in beautiful Northern Michigan. She is a nationally acclaimed travel writer. Her children are now in college.

Grandpa Larry, Larry's father, continues to live in Jonesville. He keeps busy with photography, playing the trumpet and the dogs that were given to him. Carole passed away in February, 2012. She is greatly missed.

Keri, the kid who found Heather, is … well, can't say much yet, but just keep an eye out for this girl. She has graduated from college and will be a known author in the near future.

Bev is the editor and owner of the *Breast Cancer Wellness* magazine. She is a champion for women and is changing the face of breast cancer.

Tips for Cancer Survivors and Caregivers

10 Tips for Survivors

1. Do something to kill cancer every day.
2. Gather a team that believes in you.
3. Make it a job: use schedules, determine what you need.
4. Find inspiration every day.
5. Understand your limits.
6. Sometimes it is better not to know everything.
7. Do not take care of others first. If you take the time now, you may have a lifetime to take care of loved ones again.
8. Understand that the thoughts that you have make an impact. Turn negative thoughts into positive ones.
9. Let your healthcare team know what your expectations are and what you are doing to participate in your wellness.
10. Understand that no one else is you; you are not a statistic or an outcome.

10 Tips for Caregivers

1. Be supportive, but have expectations for your survivor.
2. Let them know what you are seeing or hearing because survivors often focus on one part of a conversation and miss the rest.
3. Be open and willing to do new things. (Don't expect the same dinner as before.)
4. Keep it real—brainstorm ideas together, hash and rehash issues.
5. Help your survivor talk with doctors to clarify their ideas.
6. Be willing to let you survivor focus on themselves.
7. Research, or find someone who can muddle through information that may be beneficial to your survivor.
8. Have fun—find the cancer humor.
9. Tell your survivor that you are proud of them.
10. Help your survivor cope with changing relationships. You may have more in common with others that have cancer than your close friends.

Healing Agreement

Patient:

Recognizing that I can make a difference in healing my body, and that ultimately I am responsible for my own care, I, _____,
agree to the following:

I will be actively involved in my own care on a daily basis, making choices that will be good for my body physically, mentally and spiritually.

I will regard my treatment in a positive manner.

I will seek to have an open relationship with my healthcare providers, sharing information as to the choices I am making that could impact my medical treatment.

Healthcare Provider:

Recognizing that I can make a difference in the healing process of each patient, I, _____, agree to the following:

I recognize that my words have great influence and therefore will make every effort to be positive.

I will encourage you, my patient, to play an active role in your treatment recognizing that your efforts on a daily basis make a difference.

I will empower you to heal by acting as a partner with you in order to make informed decisions about your care.

Download a printable version at
www.EveryDayWeAreKillingCancer.com/healing-agreement

About the Author

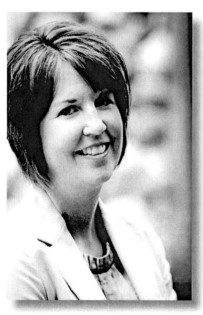

HEATHER JOSE IS an inspiring writer, speaker and columnist for Breast Cancer Wellness magazine. She is the host columnist for the Caregivers Portal [www.CaregiversPortal.com], where readers and popular writers connect with fresh ideas. She is thriving today despite a devastating diagnosis of stage IV breast cancer in her 20s. Heather is a leading advocate of facing cancer head on with family and friends, nutrition and exercise, prayer and meditation and the best of medical care. Heather travels widely as a speaker, an advocate on patient care and as the creator of Beyond Treatment Seminars.

Colophon

READ THE SPIRIT Books produces its titles using innovative digital systems that serve the emerging wave of readers who want their books delivered in a wide range of formats—from traditional print to digital readers in many shapes and sizes. This book was produced using this entirely digital process that separates the core content of the book from details of final presentation, a process that increases the flexibility and accessibility of the book's text and images. At the same time, our system ensures a well-designed, easy-to-read experience on all reading platforms, built into the digital data file itself.

David Crumm Media has built a unique production workflow employing a number of XML (Extensible Markup Language) technologies. This workflow, allows us to create a single digital "book" data file that can be delivered quickly in all formats from traditionally bound print-on-paper to nearly any digital reader you care to choose, including Amazon Kindle®, Apple iBook®, Barnes and Noble Nook® and other devices that support the ePub and PDF digital book formats.

And due to the efficient "print-on-demand" process we use for printed books, we invite you to visit us online to learn more about opportunities to order quantities of this book with the possibility of personalizing a "group read" for your organization or congregation by putting your organizations logo and name on the cover of the copies you order. You can even add your own introductory pages to this book for your church or organization.

During production, we use Adobe InDesign®, <Oxygen/>® XML Editor and Microsoft Word® along with custom tools built in-house.

The print edition is set in Minion Pro and Myrias Pro.

Cover art and Design by Rick Nease: www.RickNeaseArt.com.

Editing by Kathy MacDonald.

Copy editing and XML styling by Celeste Dykas.

Digital encoding and print layout by John Hile.

If you enjoyed this book, you may also enjoy

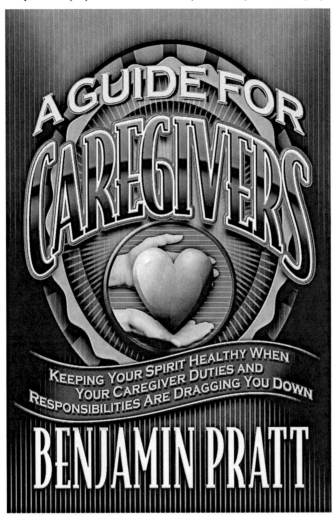

In one out of three households, someone is a caregiver: women and men who give of body, mind and soul to care for the well being of others. They need daily, practical help in reviving their spirits and avoiding burnout.

http://www.GuideForCaregivers.com

ISBN: 978-1-934879-27-6

If you enjoyed this book, you may also enjoy

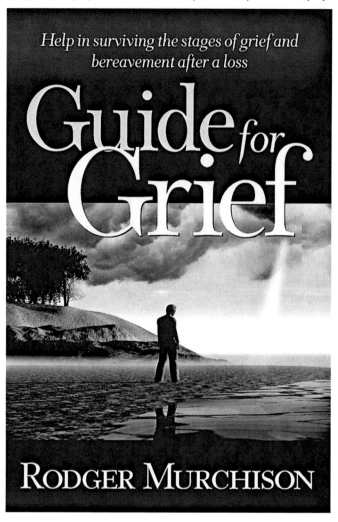

Help in surviving the stages of grief and
bereavement after a loss

Guide for
Grief

RODGER MURCHISON

In his new Guide for Grief, the Rev. Rodger Murchison
brings years of pastoral experience and study, sharing
recommendations from both scripture and the latest
research into loss and bereavement.

http://www.GuideForGrief.com

ISBN: 978-1-934879-31-3

If you enjoyed this book, you may also enjoy

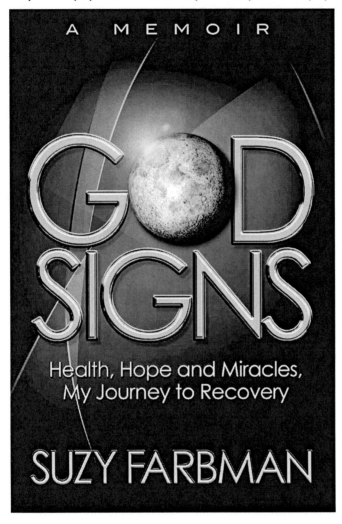

Suzy Farbman has entertained millions of readers throughout her career as a writer. You're in the hands of a wise, often funny and startlingly honest friend in the pages of her books.

http://www.GodsignsBook.com

ISBN: 978-1-934879-58-0

CPSIA information can be obtained at www.ICGtesting.com
Printed in the USA
BVOW070430011012

301703BV00006B/4/P